Give It a Go, Eat a Rainbow

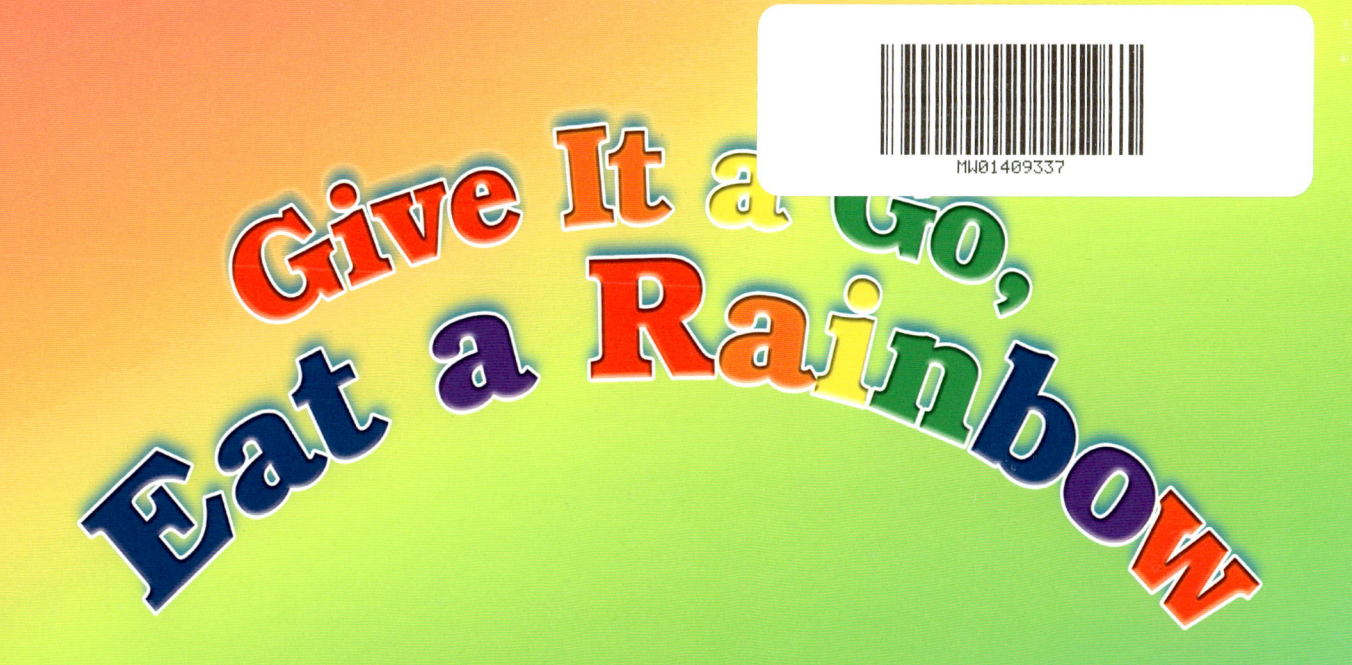

Written by
Kathryn Kemp Guylay

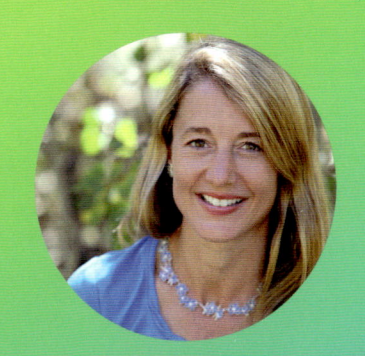

Illustrated by
Alexander Guylay

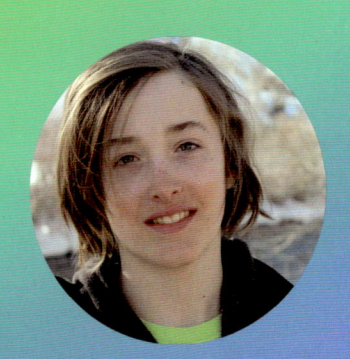

1

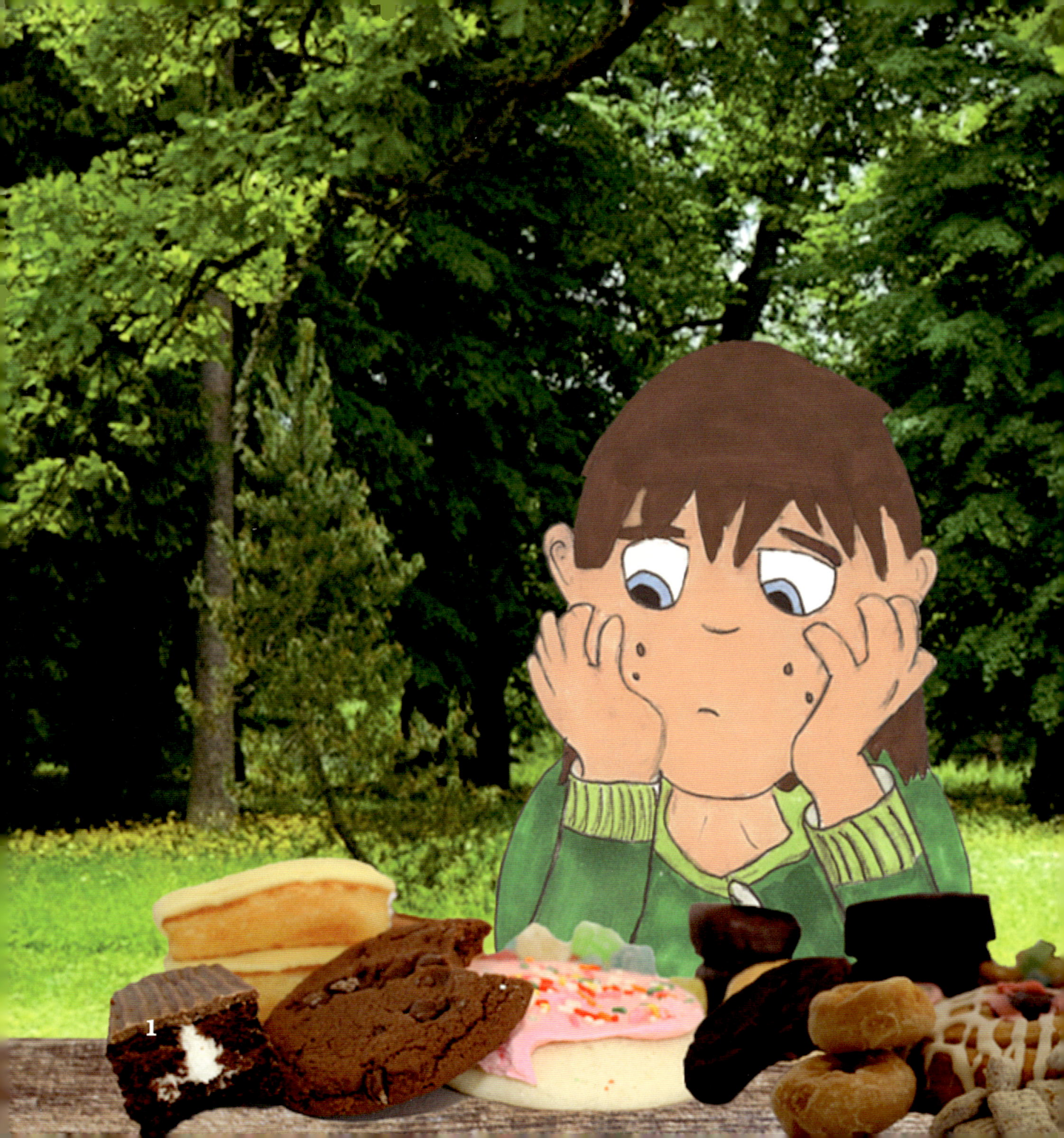

MEET **BLAKE.** Blake is sleepy.

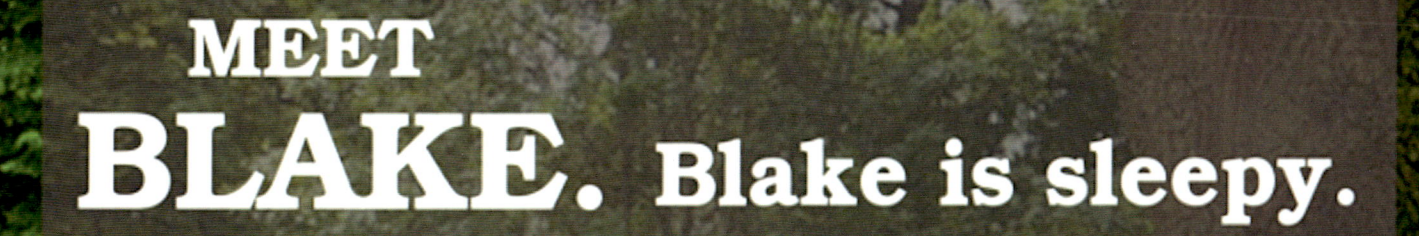

Blake's tummy hurts;
it makes Blake weepy.

Cake is all Blake likes to eat;
cookies, candies
- all things sweet.

Why do I feel so. . .slow, when other kids can go, Go, GO?

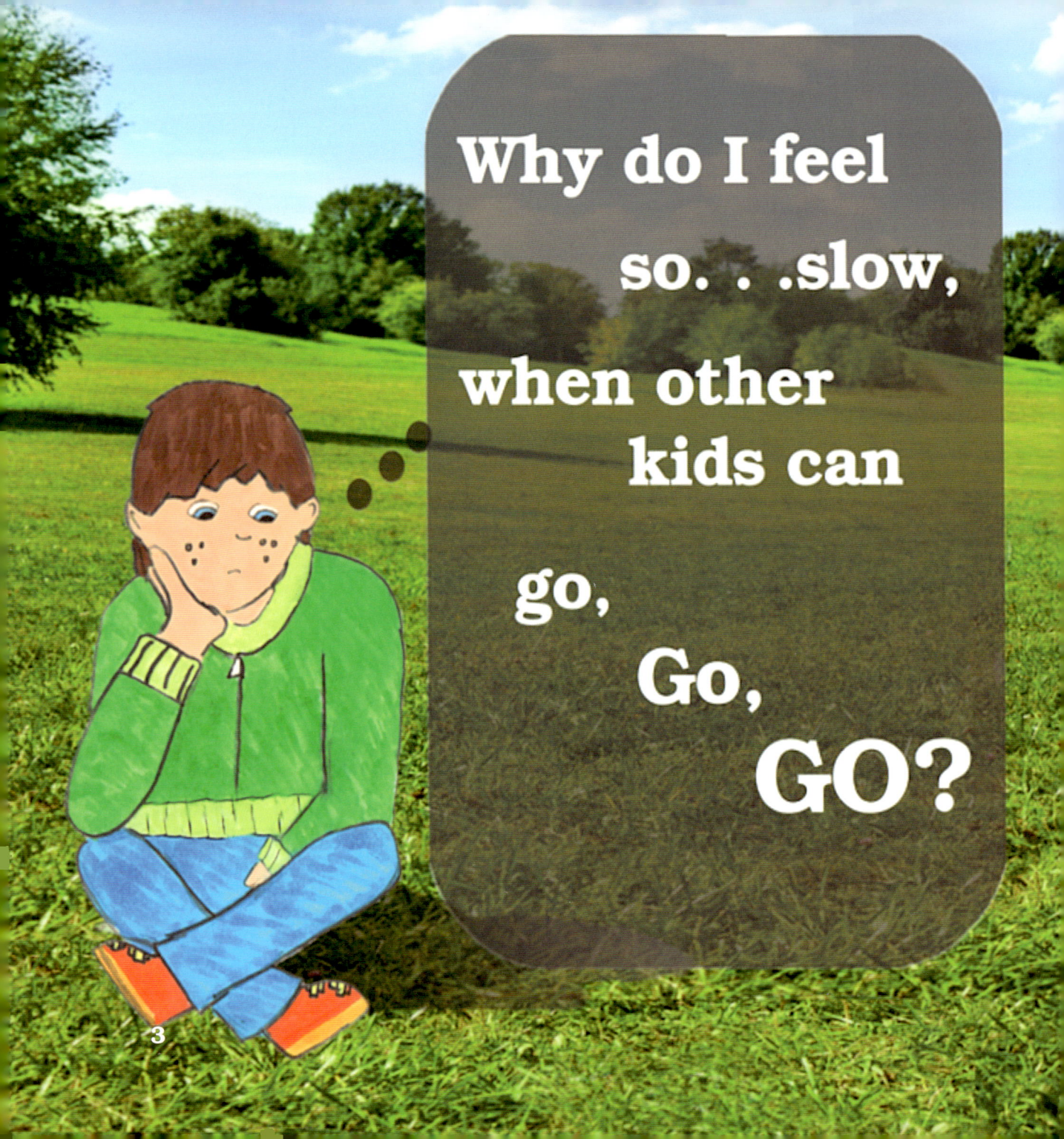

4

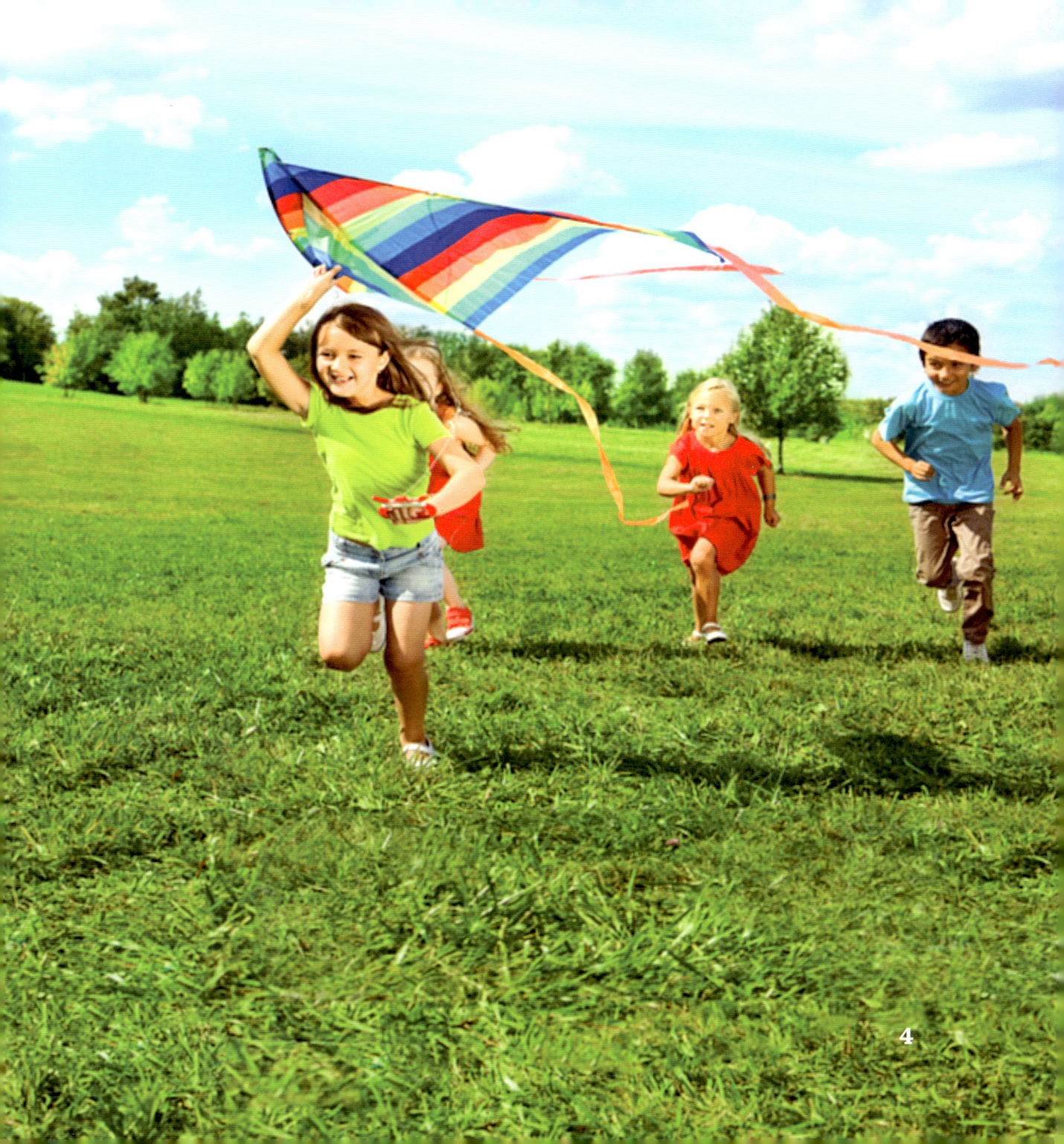

One day,
just around
the bend,

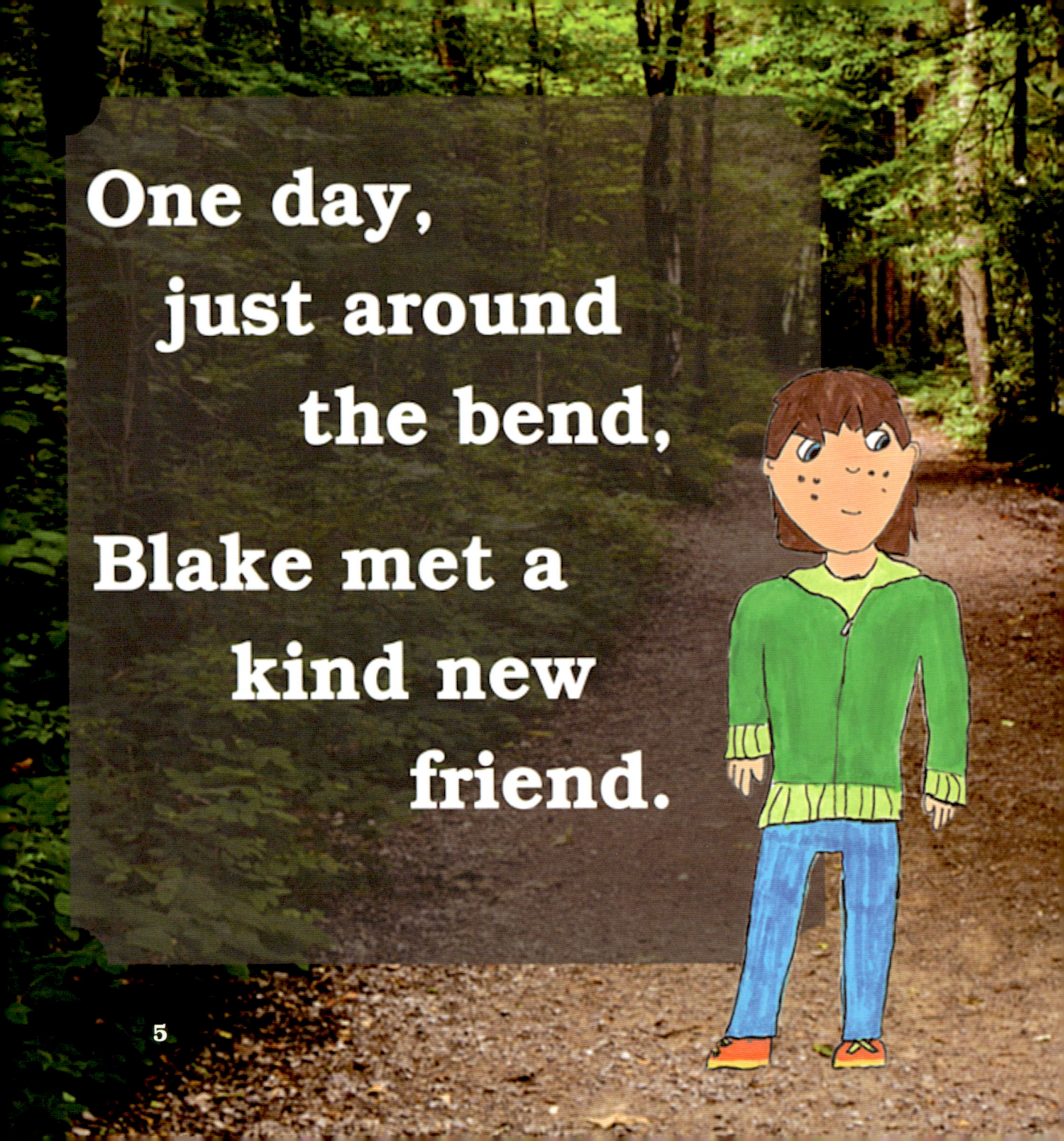

Blake met a
kind new
friend.

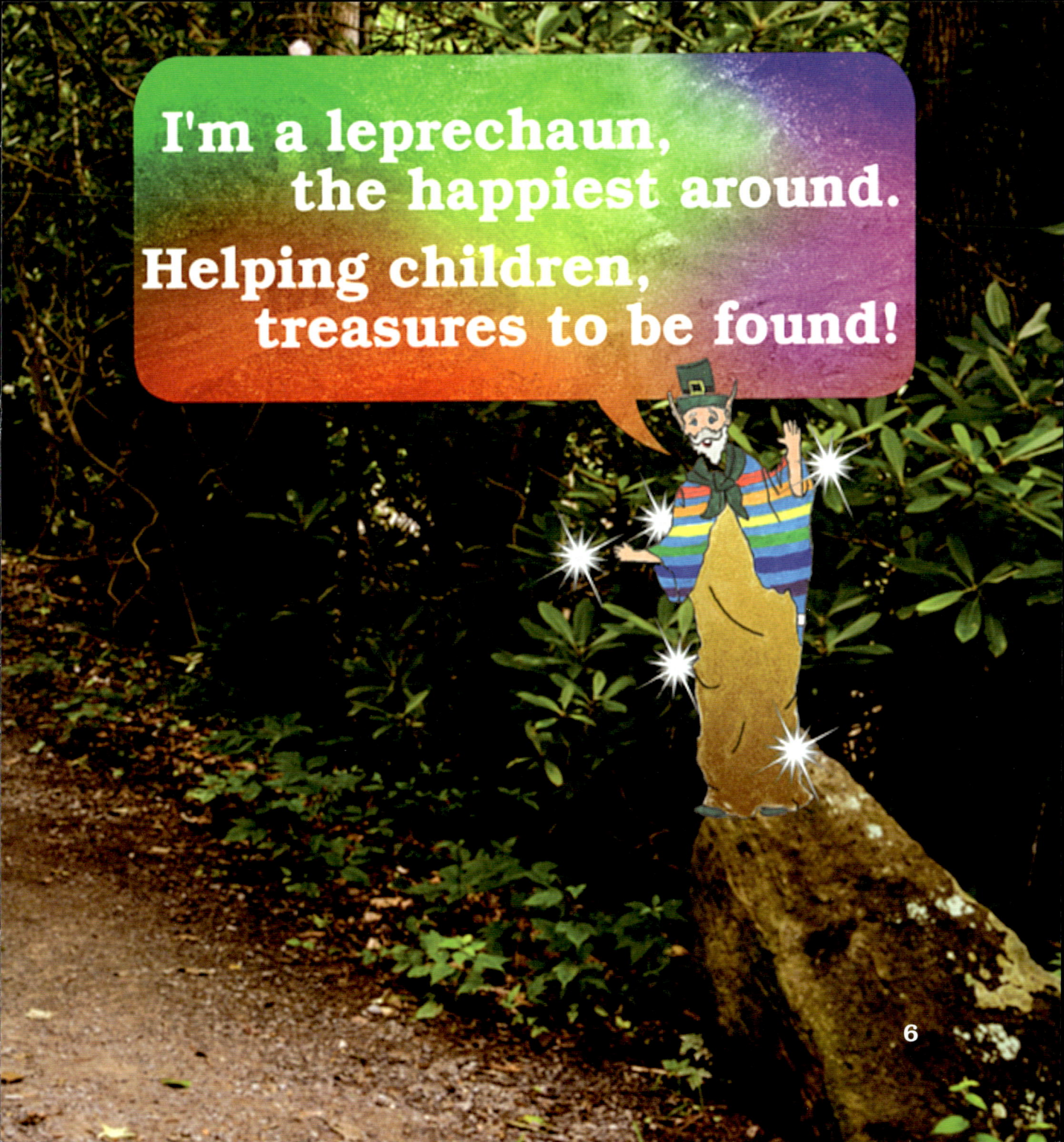

I'm a leprechaun,
    the happiest around.
Helping children,
    treasures to be found!

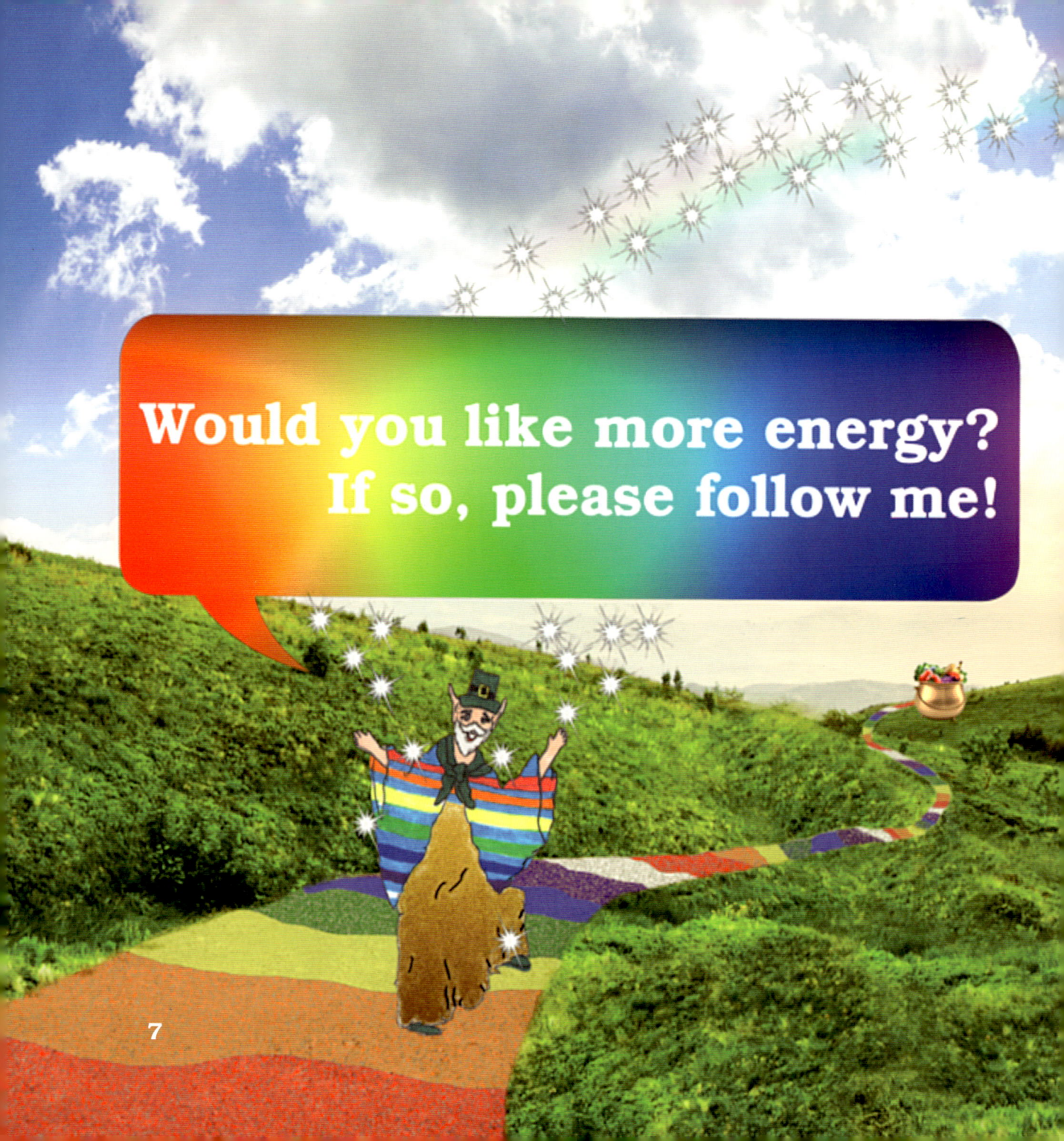

**Would you like more energy?
If so, please follow me!**

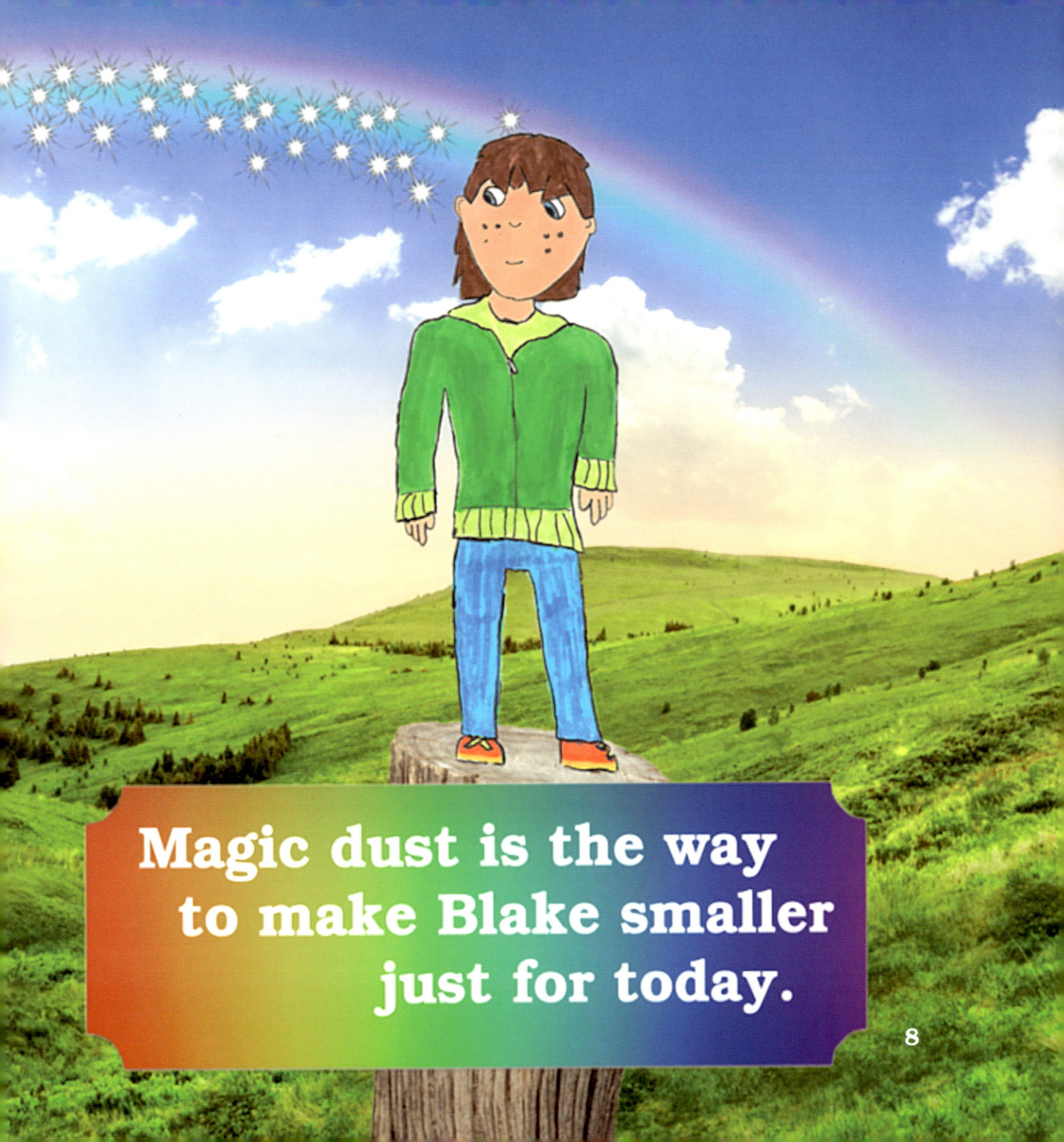

Magic dust is the way to make Blake smaller just for today.

9

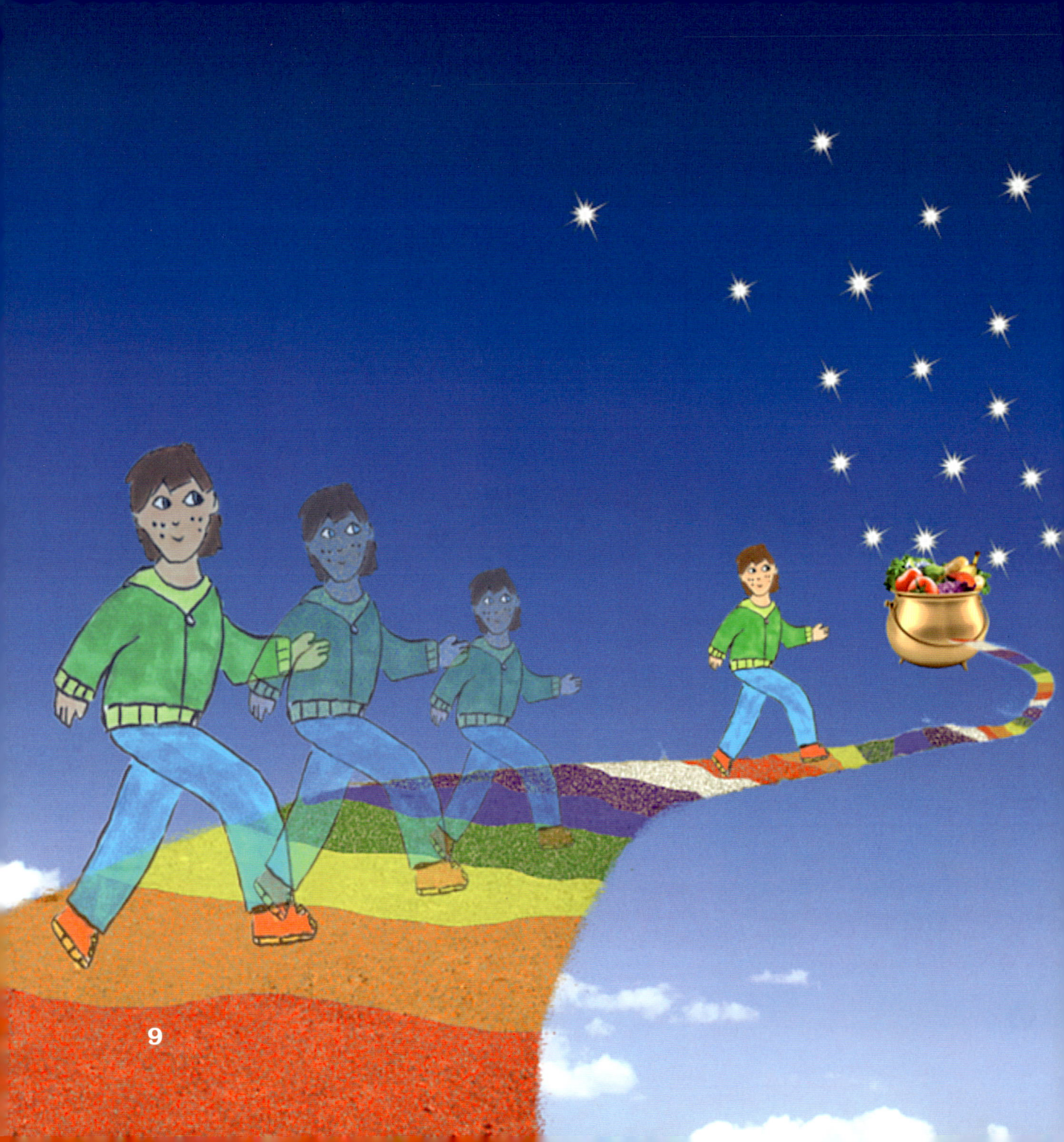

Have fun
and give it a go!
Time to
follow the rainbow.

Every color in the
rainbow is key,
to find the pot of gold,
you'll see!

11

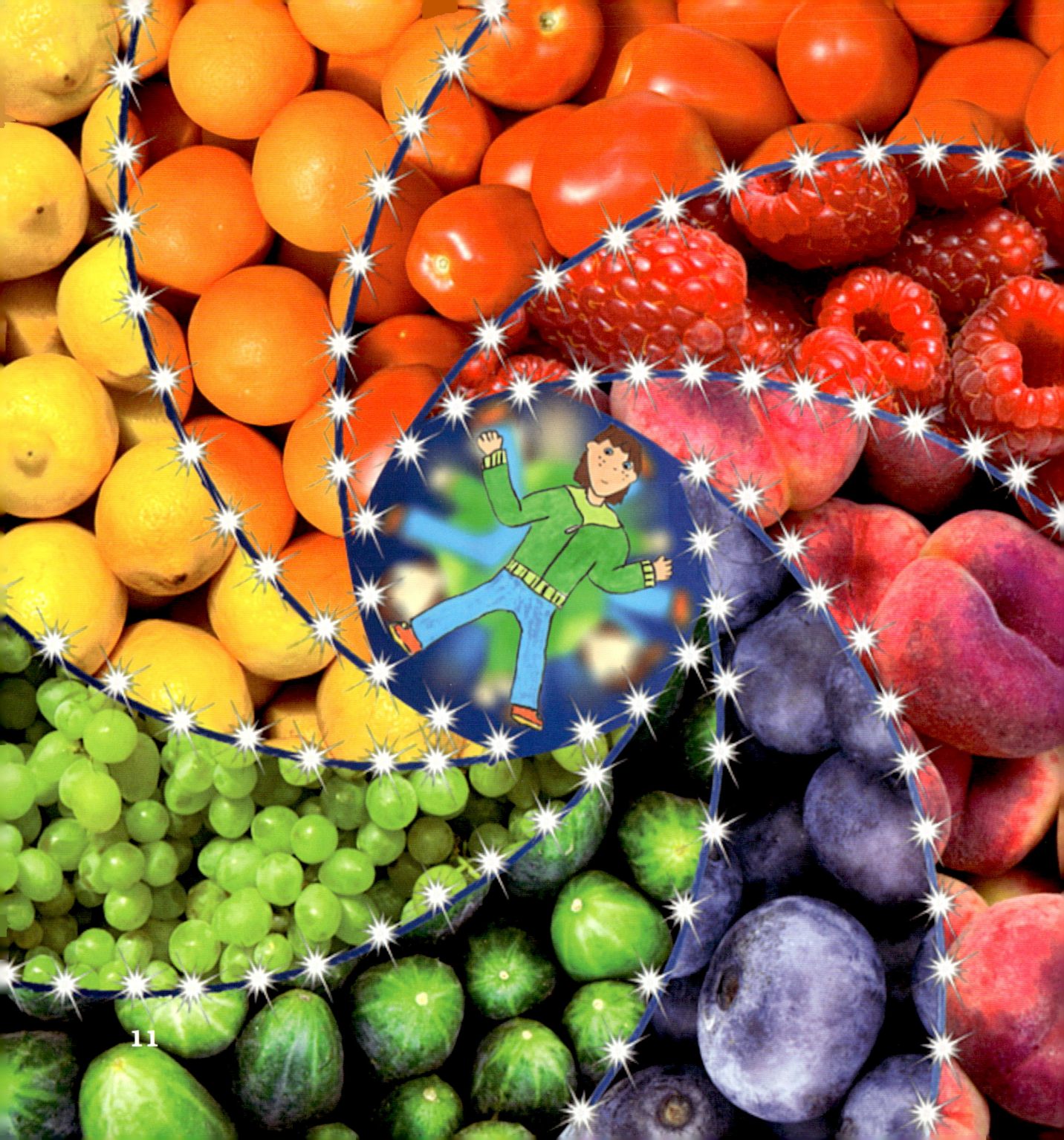

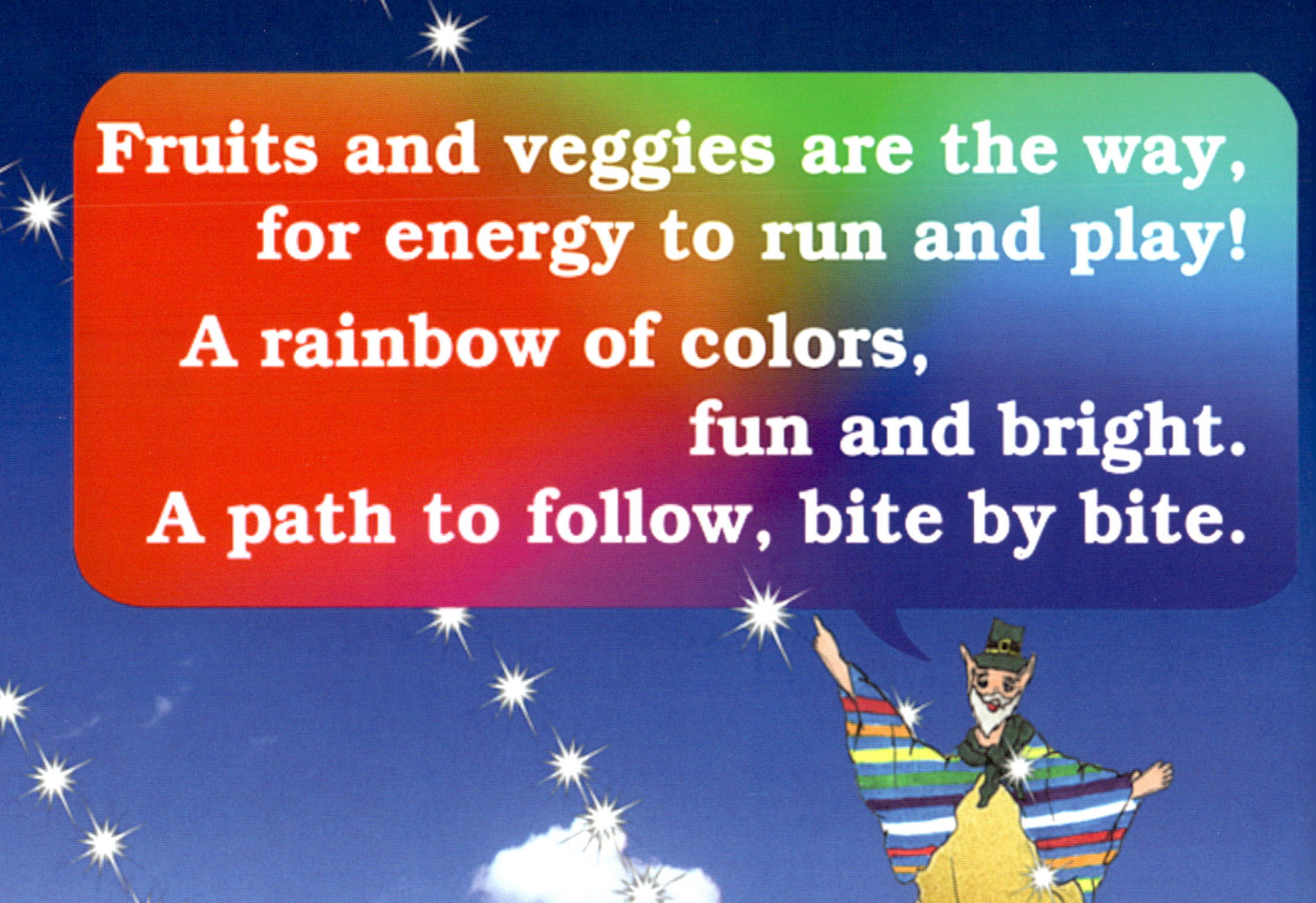

Fruits and veggies are the way,
for energy to run and play!
A rainbow of colors,
fun and bright.
A path to follow, bite by bite.

RED is where your journey will start.

RED is very good for your heart.

? What red food is shown to the right?
ANSWER: Tomatoes

That food is good for Blake's _____.
ANSWER: Heart

14

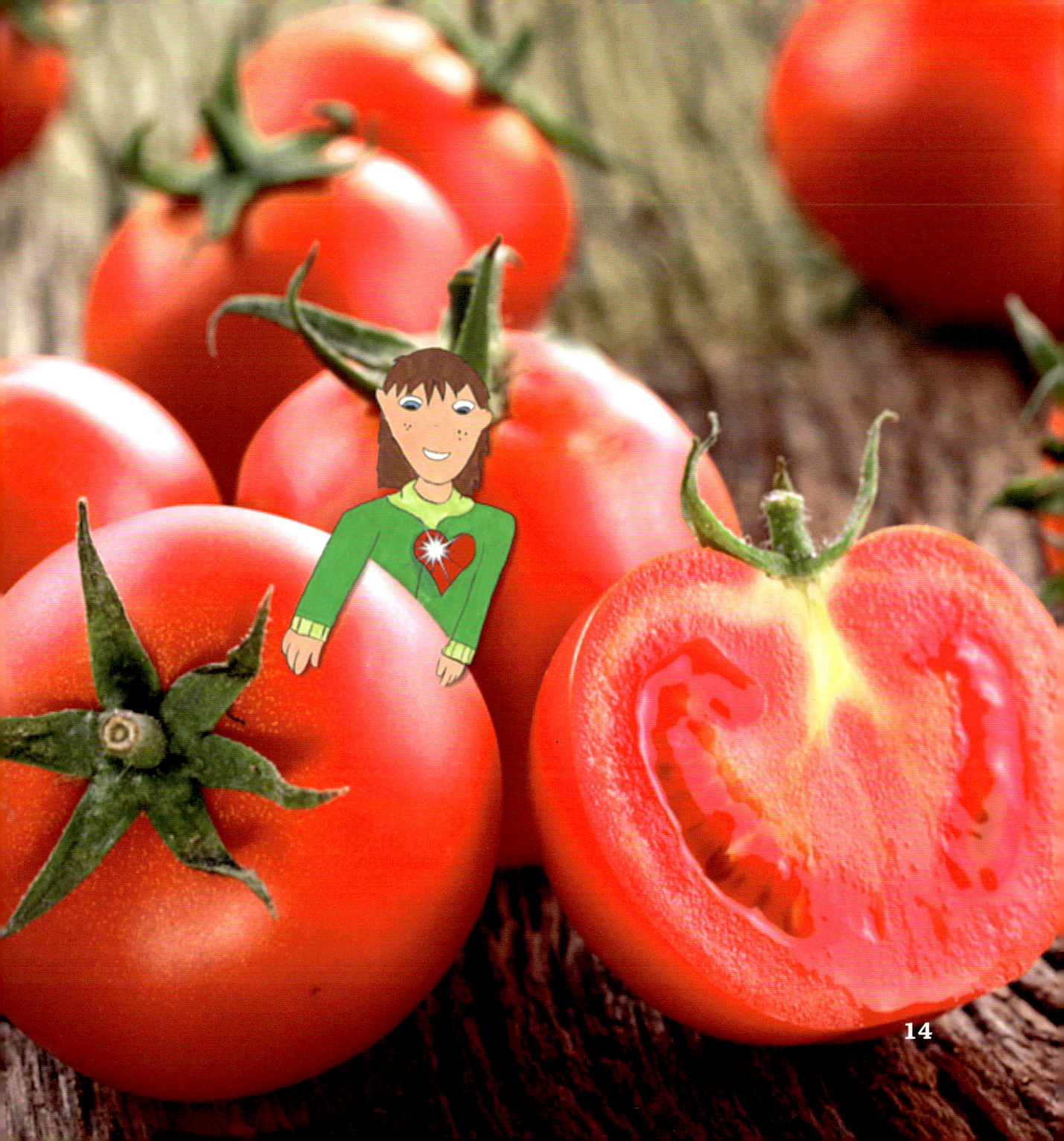

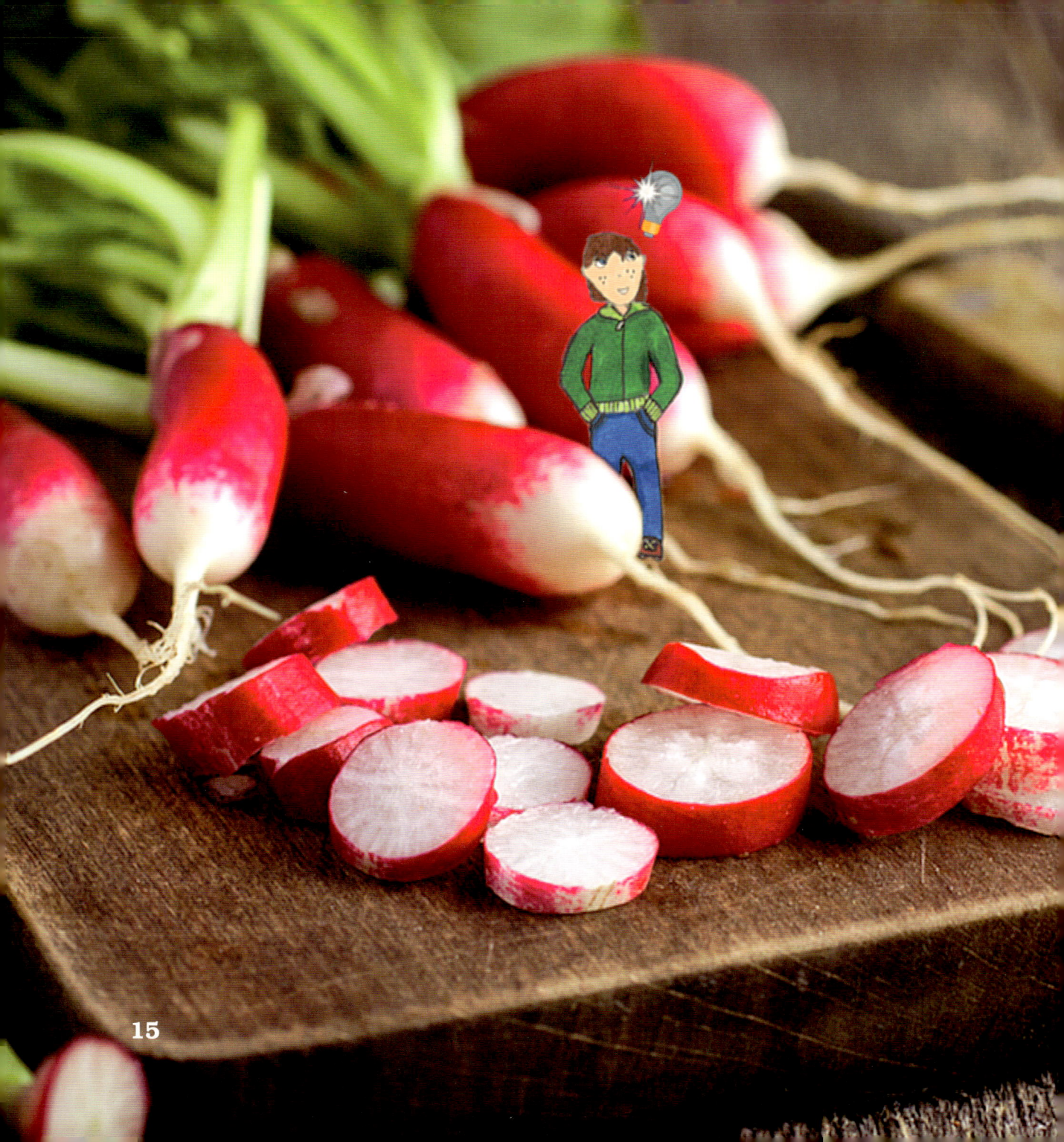

Inside RED fruits and veggies you'll find nutrients so very good for your mind.

? **What red veggies are shown to the left?**
ANSWER: Radishes

Those veggies are good for Blake's _____.
ANSWER: Brain

[?] **What are some other RED fruits and veggies?**

ANSWER: Cherry, strawberries, raspberries, red pepper

[?] **Do you want to help Blake reach the pot of gold?**

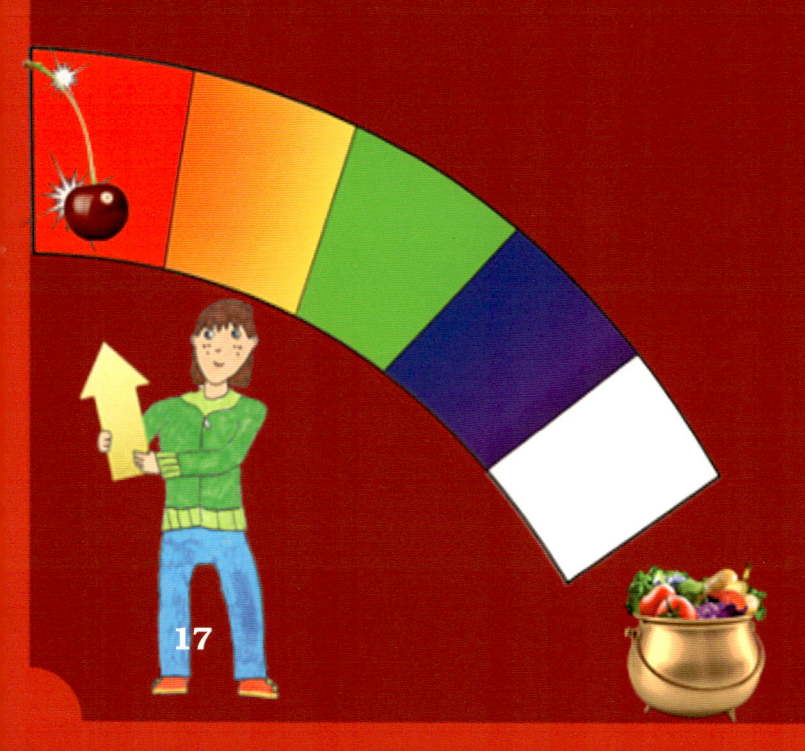

18

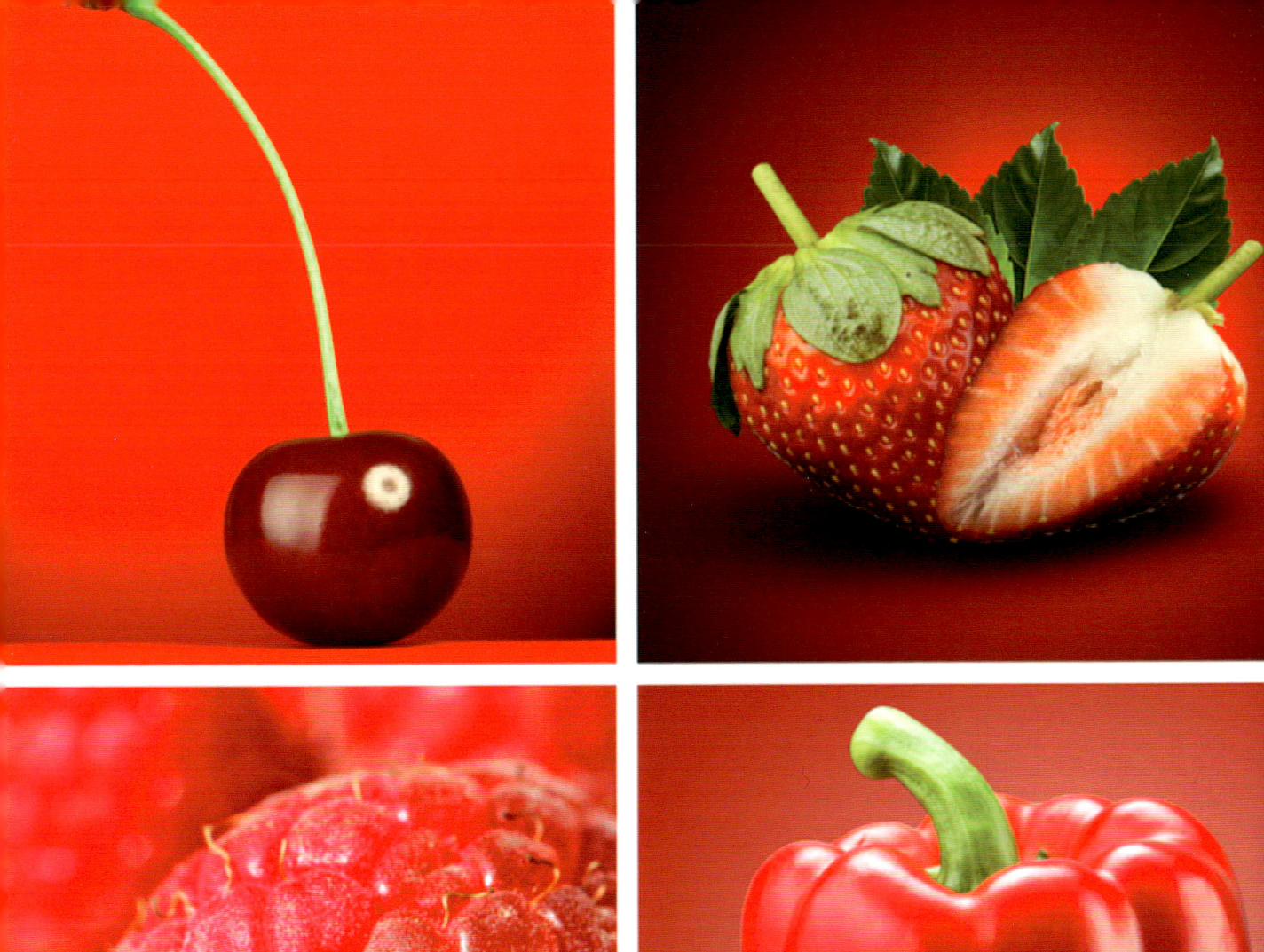

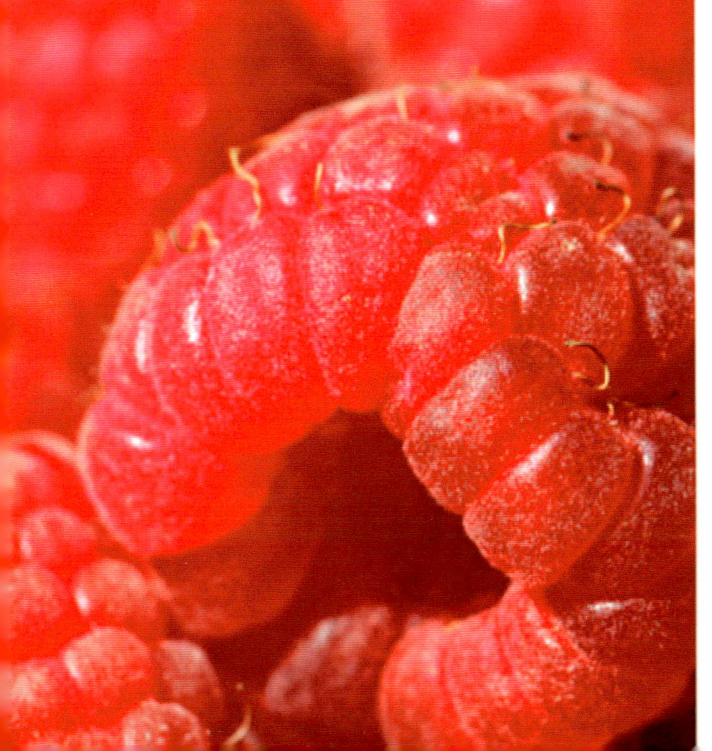

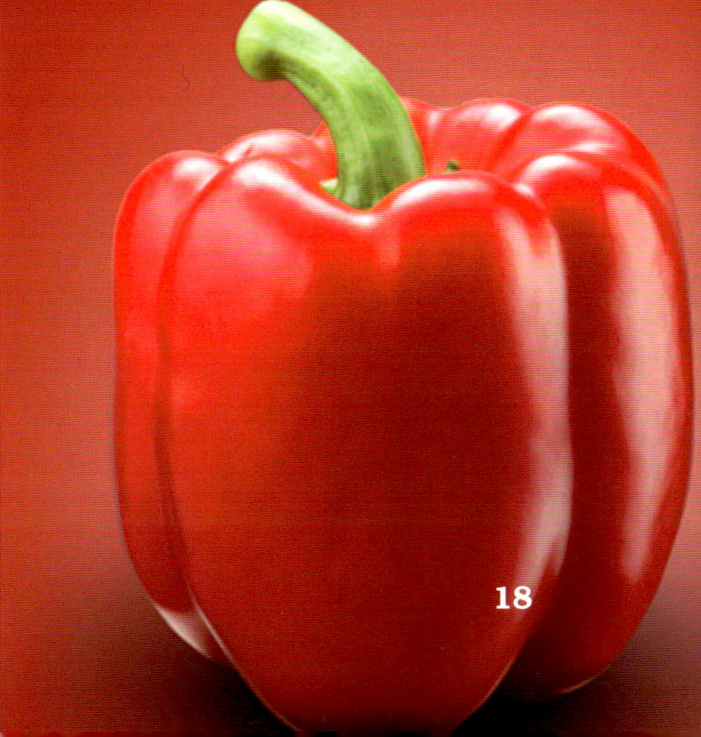

19

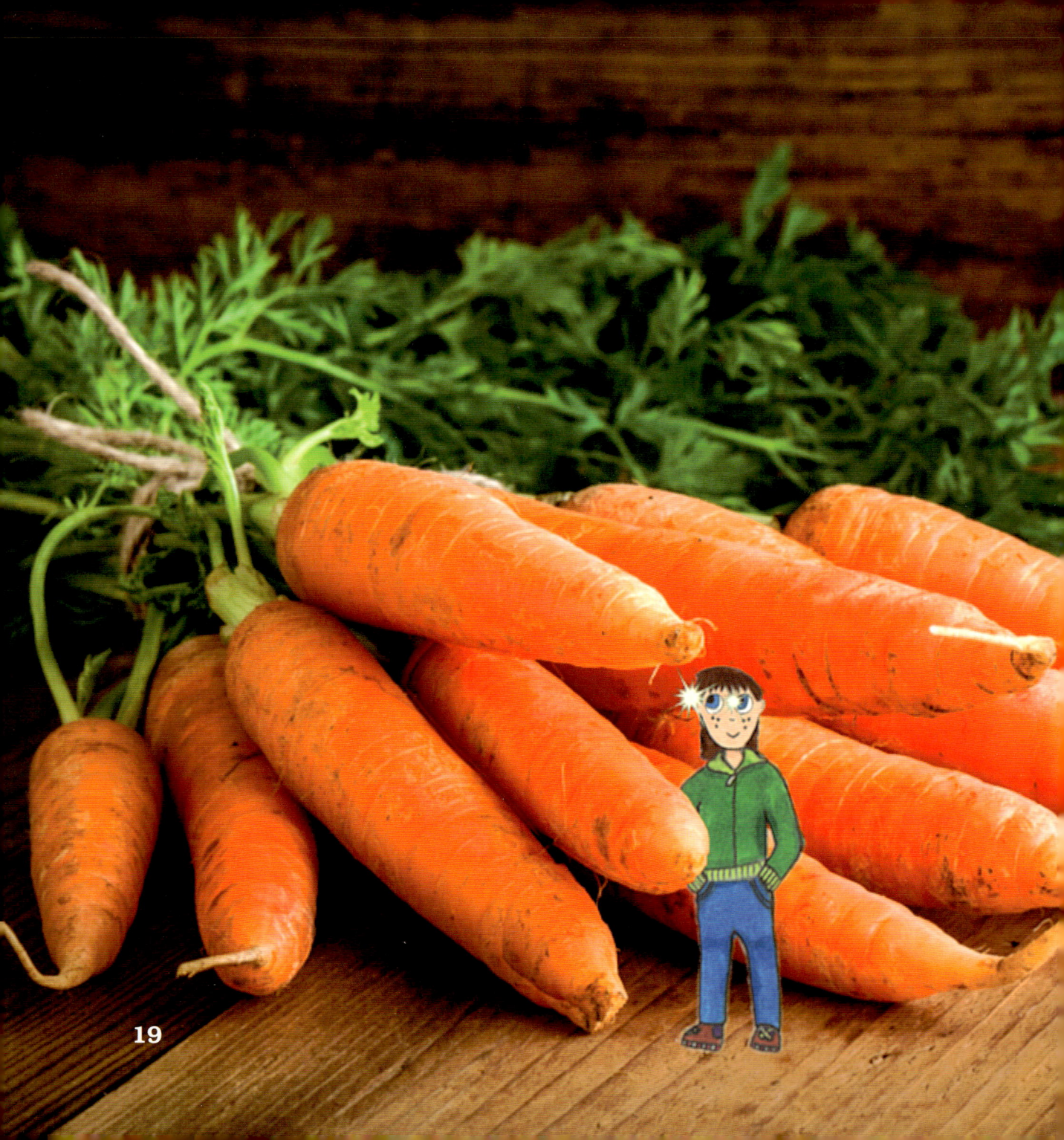

Let's move ahead with precision.

ORANGE and YELLOW help your vision.

? What orange veggies are shown to the left?
ANSWER: Carrots

Those veggies are good for Blake's _____.
ANSWER: Eyes

We're getting closer to the pot of gold. Eat **ORANGE** and **YELLOW** to avoid a cold!

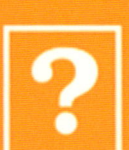

? What yellow fruit is shown to the right?
ANSWER: Pineapple

That fruit is good for Blake's _____.
ANSWER: Strength

22

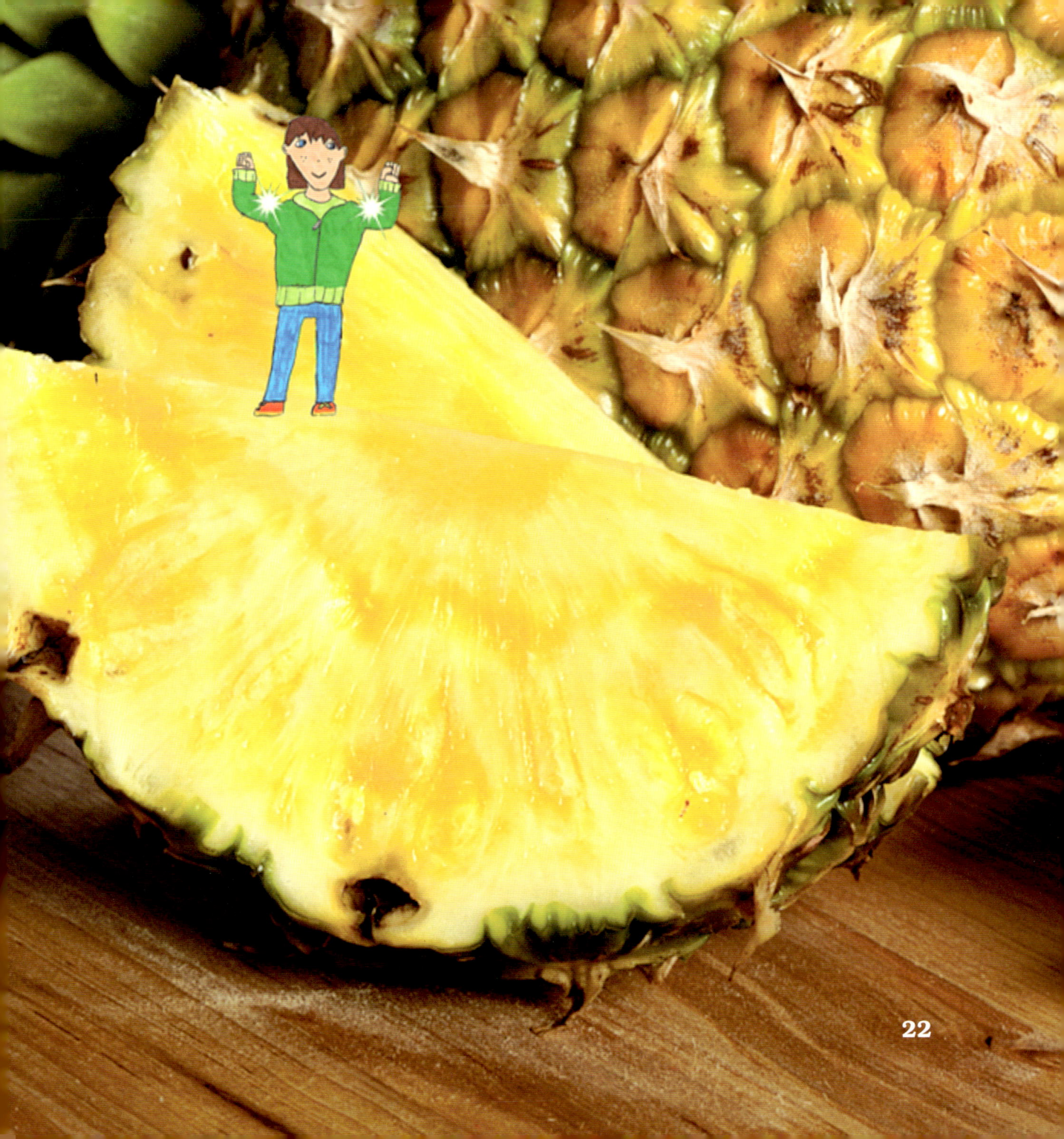

23

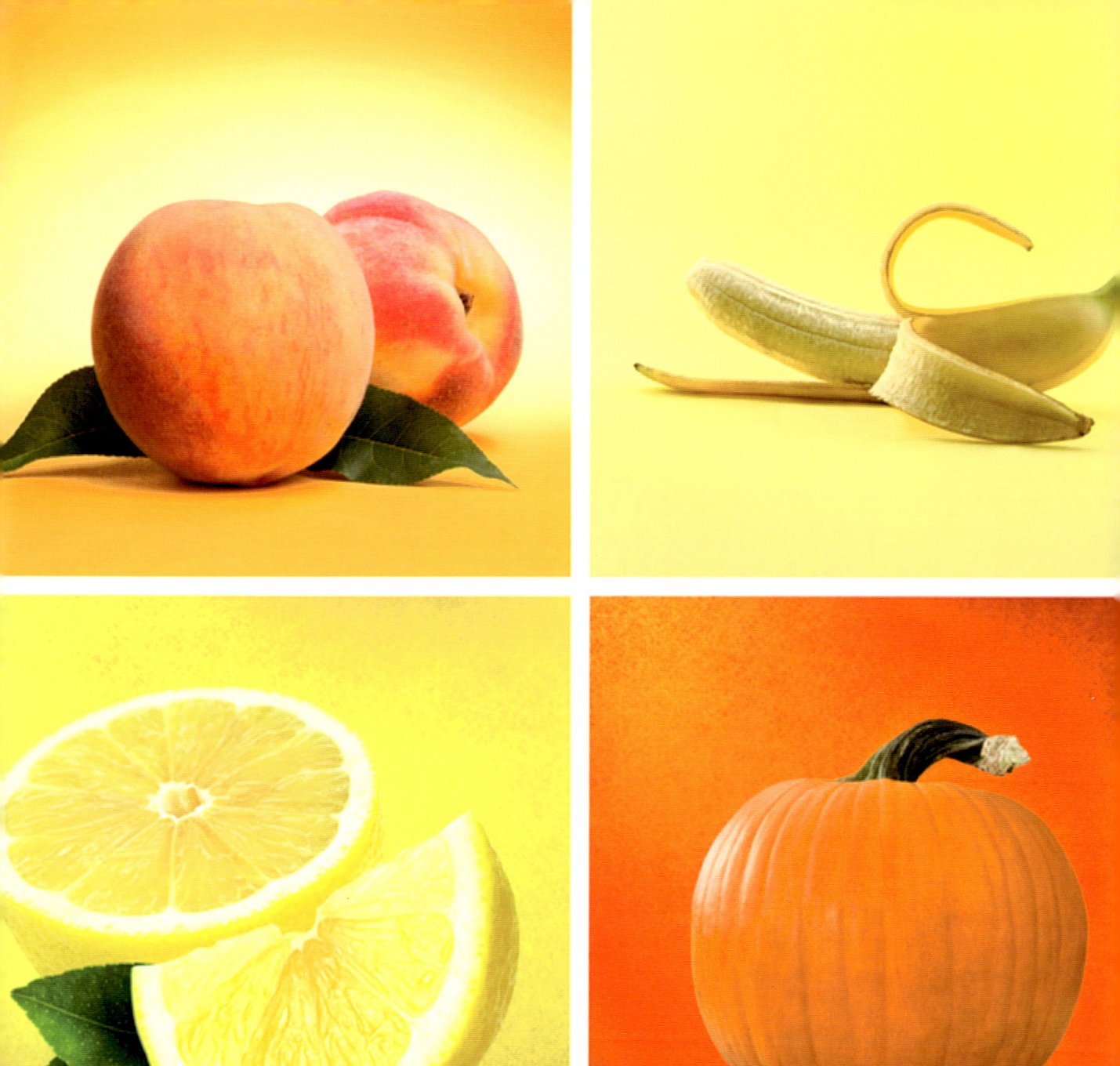

? **What are some other ORANGE and YELLOW fruits and veggies?**

ANSWER: Peaches, banana, lemon, pumpkin

? **How many color steps left until we reach the pot of gold?**

ANSWER: Three

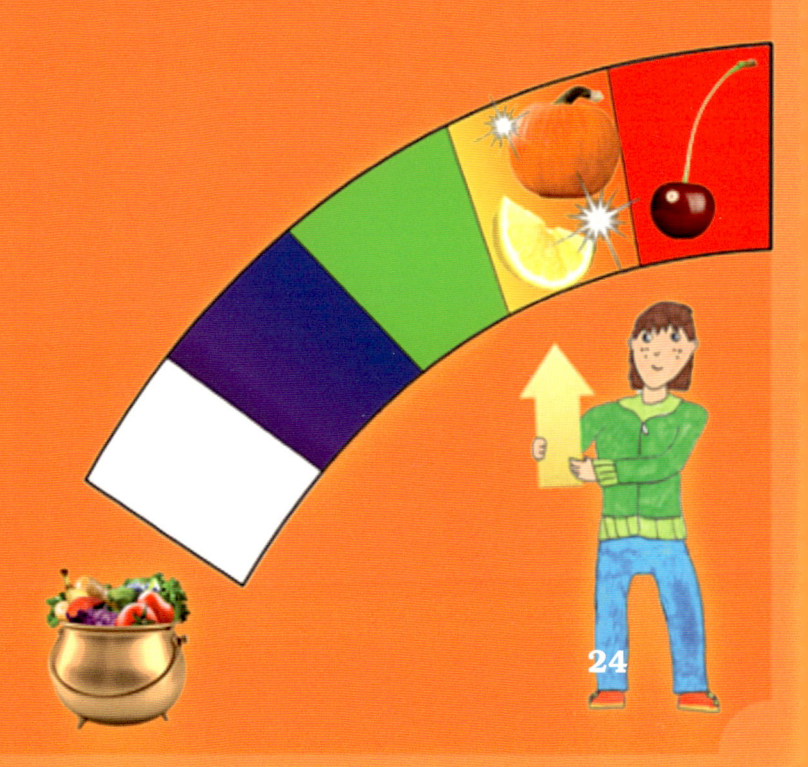

Treasures await,
you'll see what I mean!
Your teeth and bones
get strong with
GREEN.

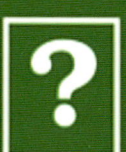

? **What green veggie is shown to the right?**
ANSWER: Broccoli

That veggie is good for Blake's _____ .
ANSWER: Teeth

26

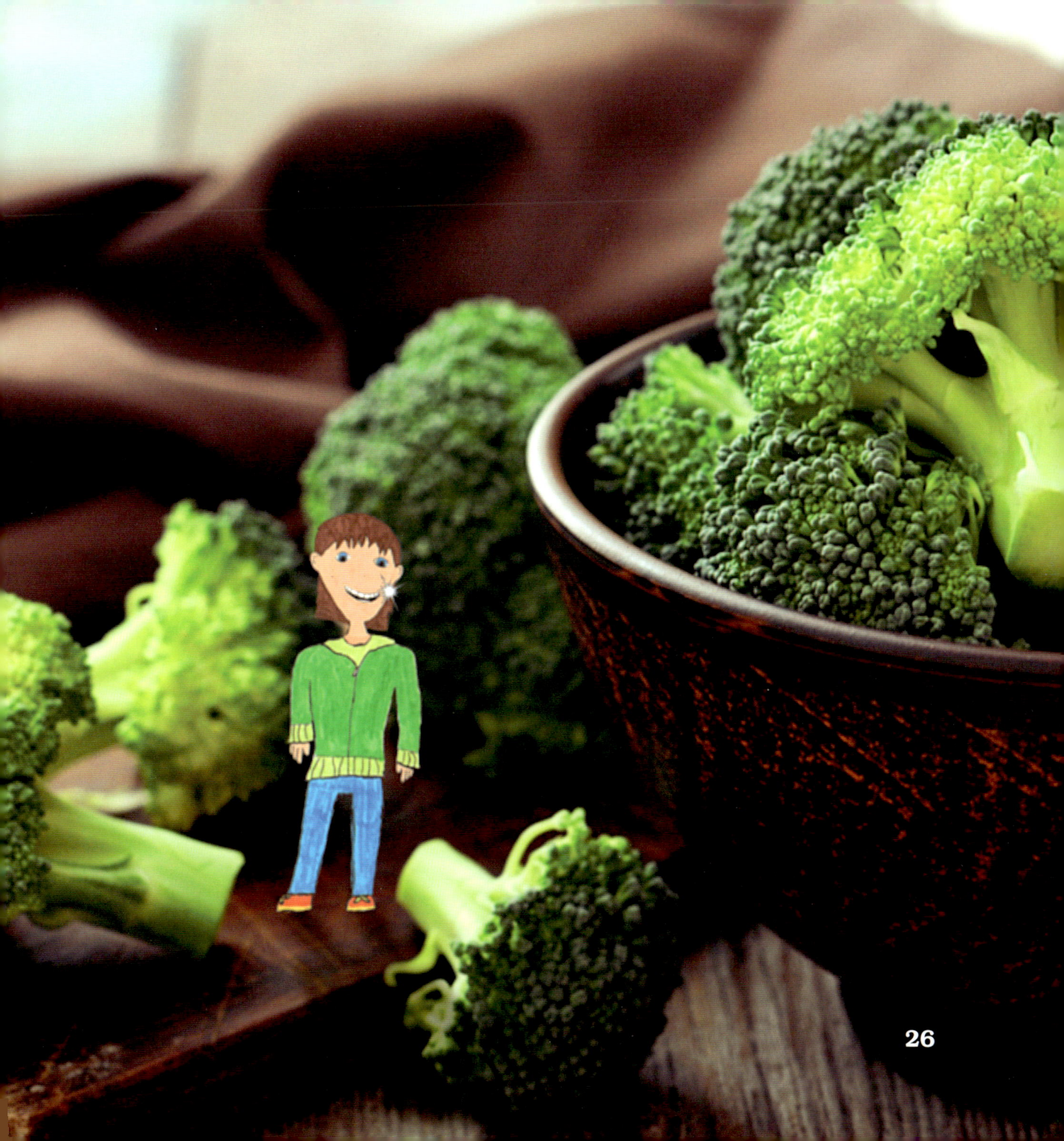

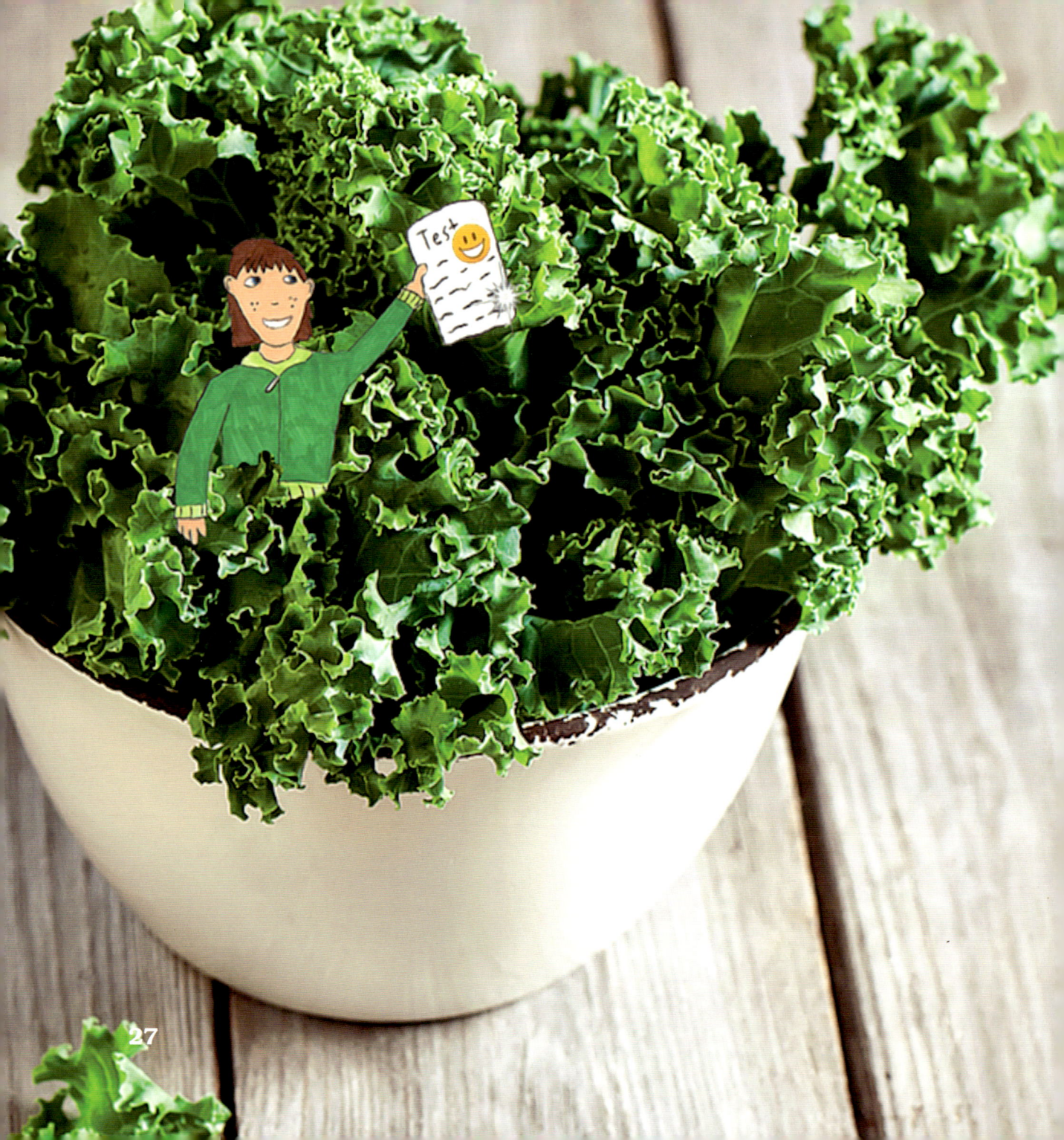

Calcium is found in spinach and kale. Eat GREEN foods, and you won't fail!

? What green veggie is shown to the left?
ANSWER: Kale

How is Blake doing in school thanks to eating green veggies?
ANSWER: Great!

? **What are some other GREEN fruits and veggies?**

ANSWER: Brussels sprouts, asparagus, kiwi, celery

? **How many color steps left to reach the pot of gold?**

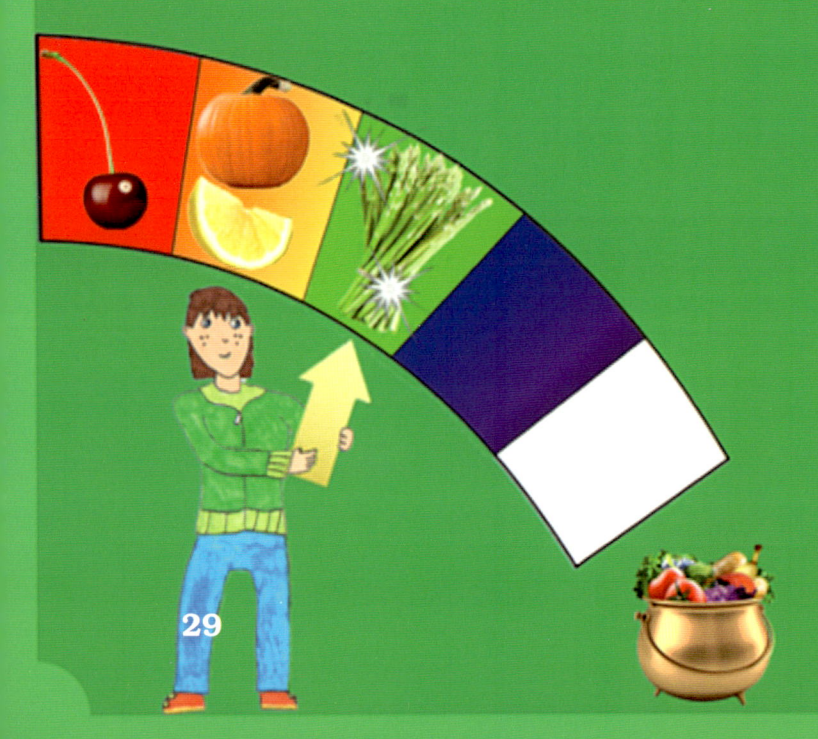

ANSWER: Two!

30

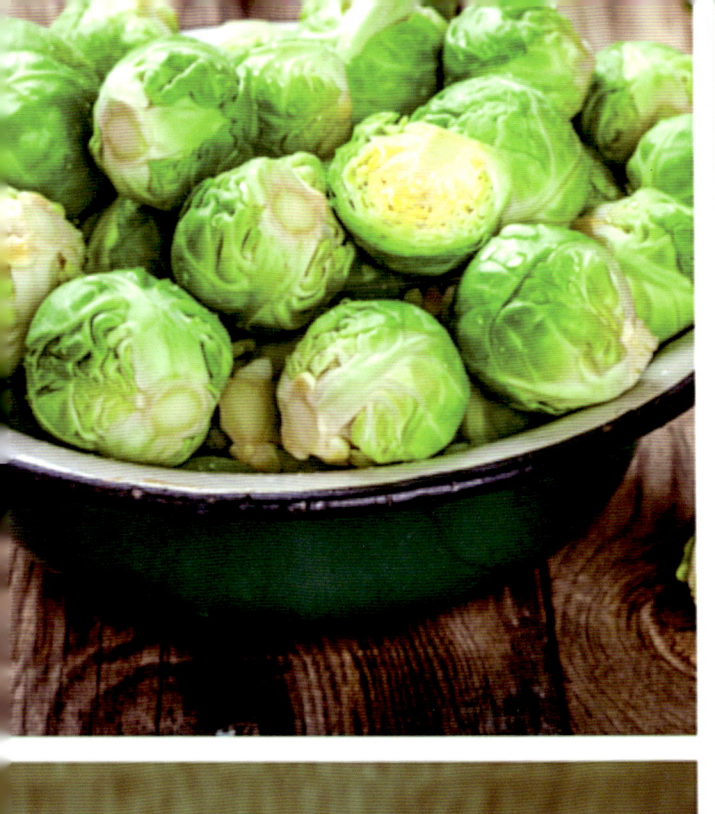

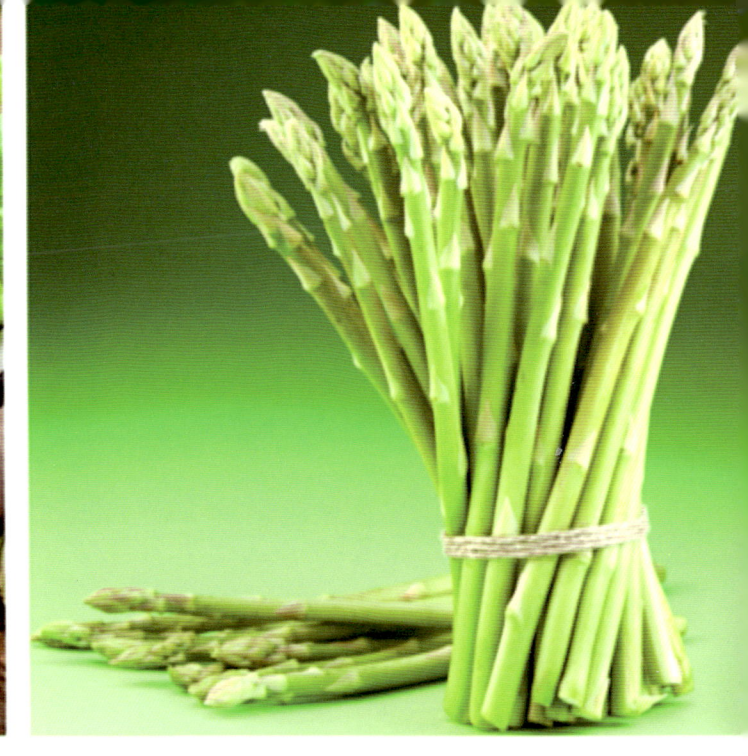

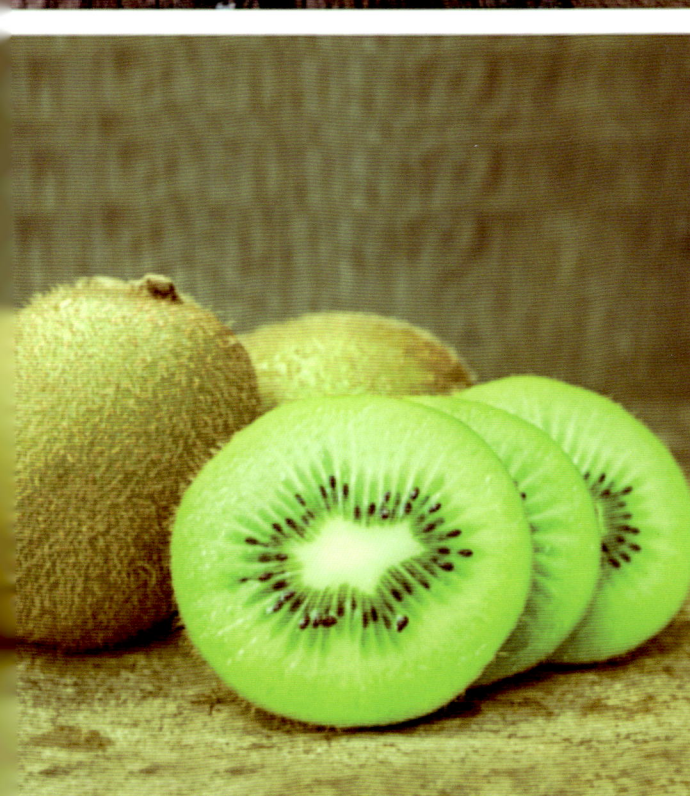

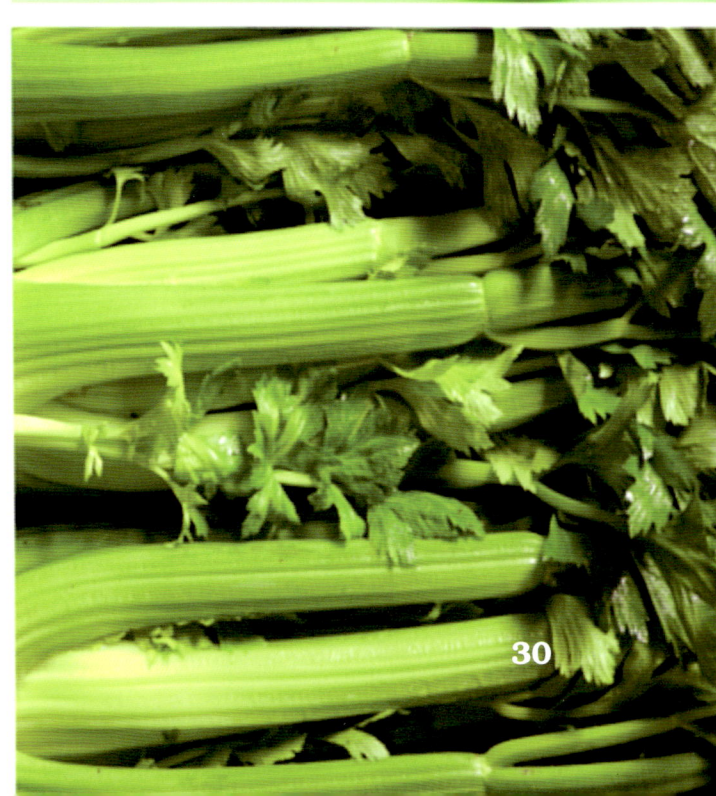

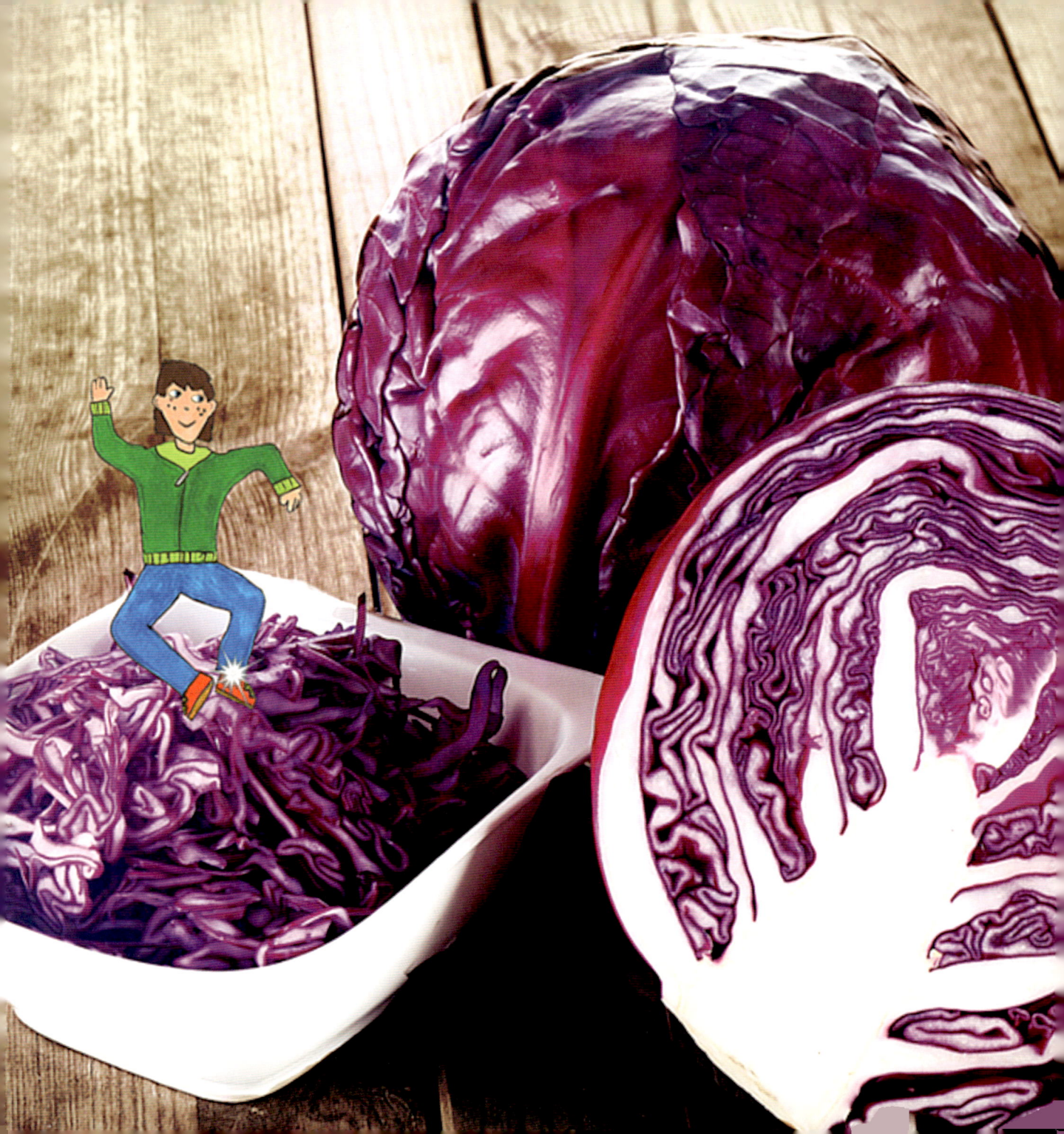

BLUE and PURPLE

– our next step.
Eating these foods
will give you pep!

? What purple veggie is shown to the left?
ANSWER: Purple cabbage

That veggie is good for Blake's _____.
ANSWER: Energy

Want to run fast and free?
BLUE and PURPLE give you energy!

What blue fruits are shown to the right?
ANSWER: Blueberries

Those fruits are good for Blake's _____.
ANSWER: Speed

34

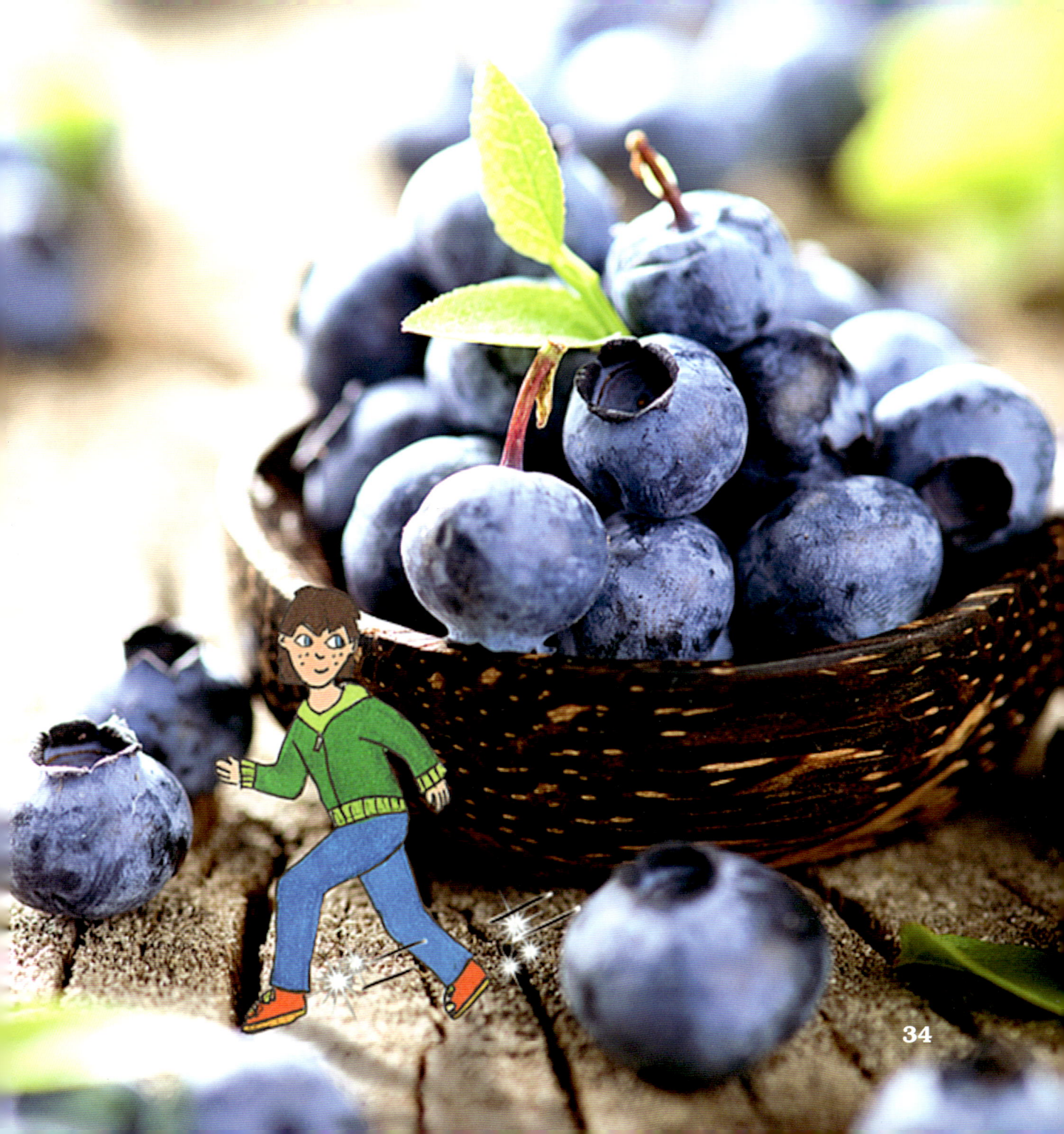

35

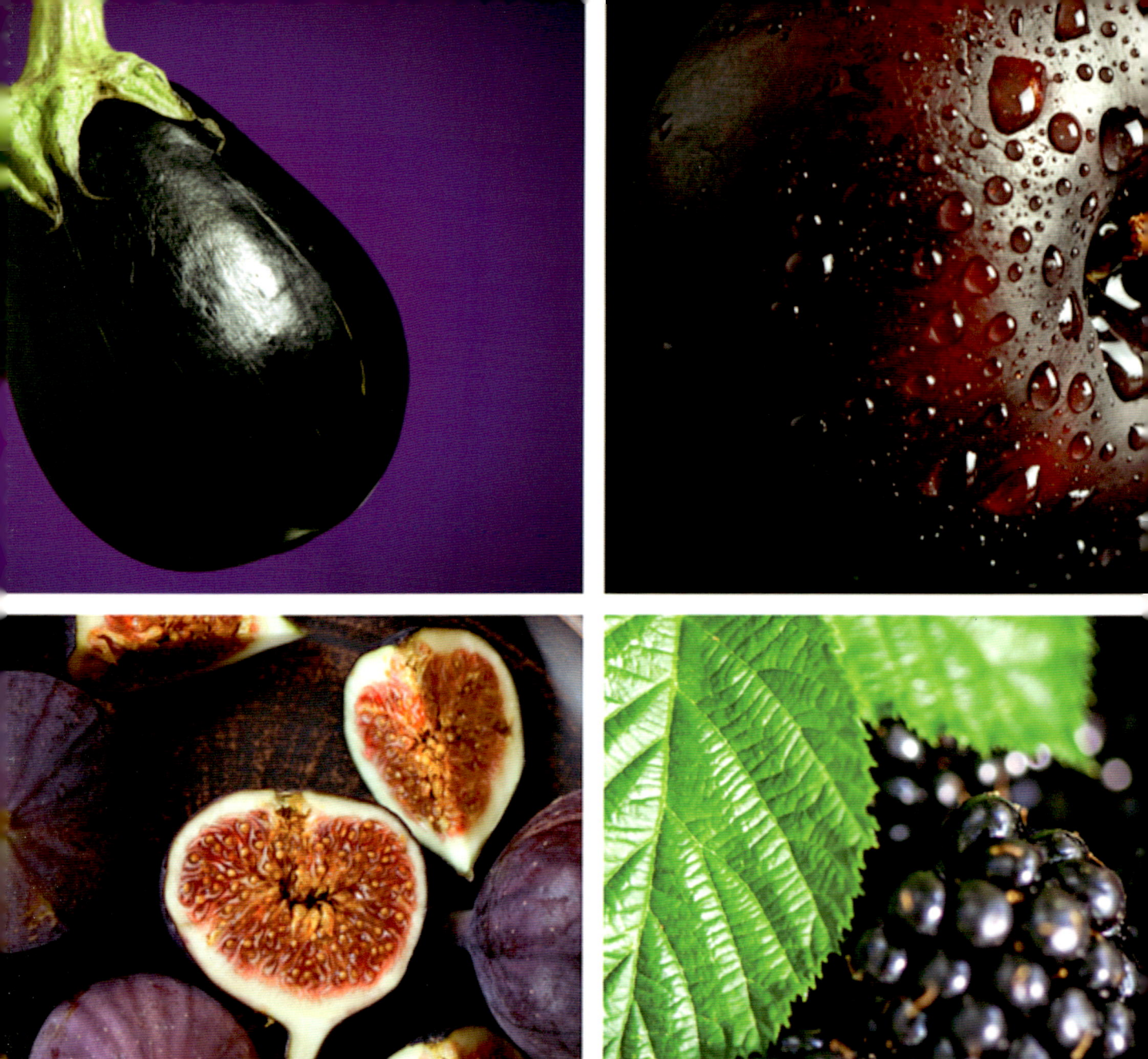

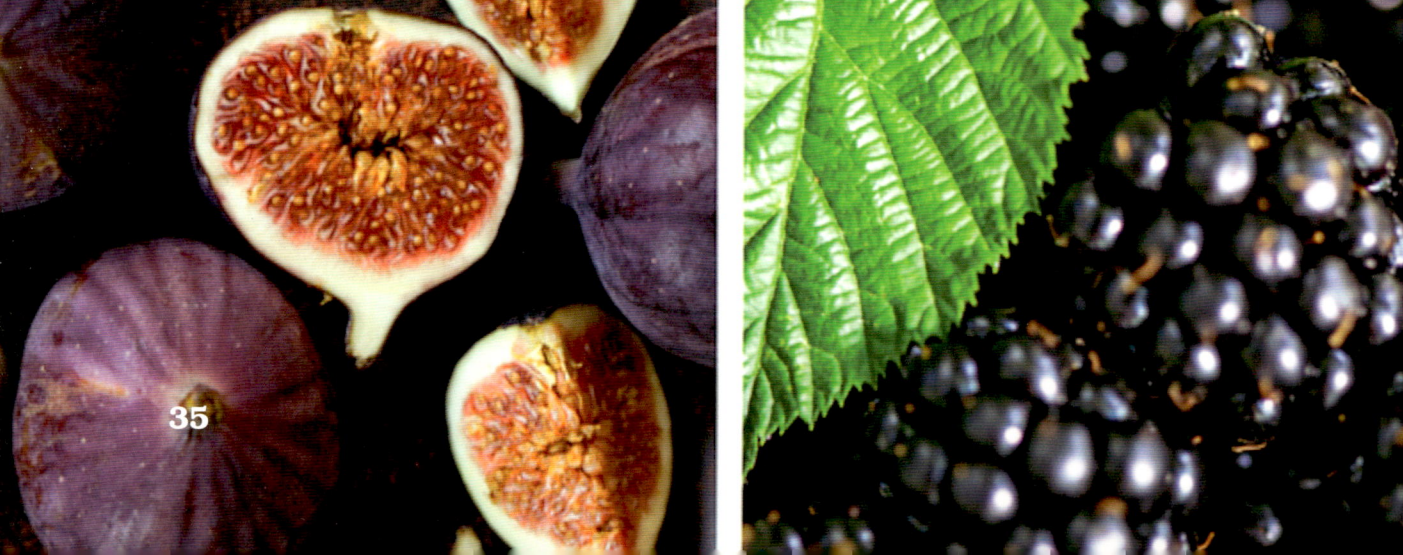

? What are some other **BLUE** and **PURPLE** fruits and veggies?

ANSWER: Eggplant, plum, figs, blackberries

? How many color steps left until we reach the pot of gold?

ANSWER: Only one!

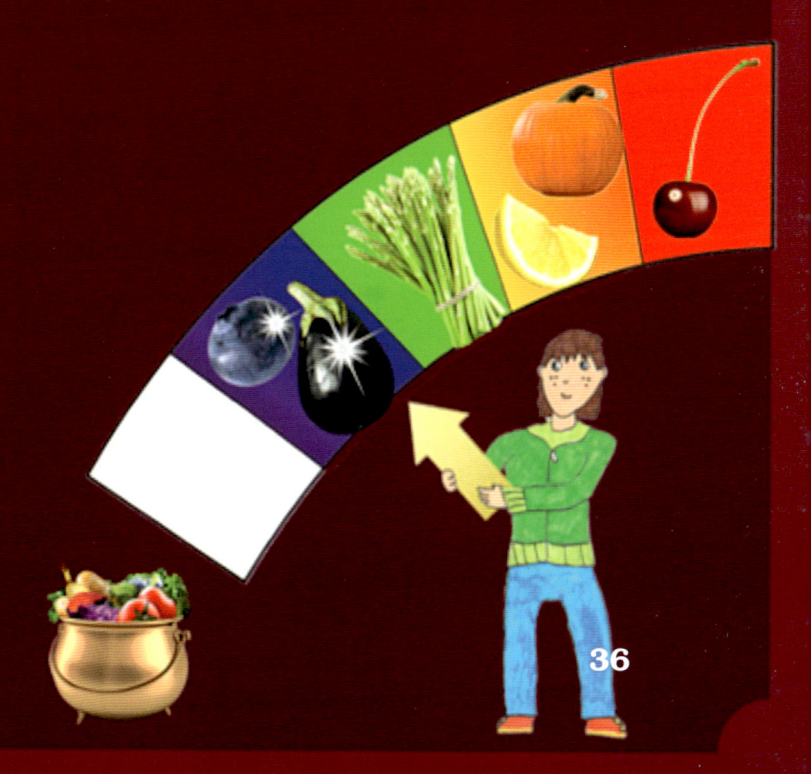

The last color on our path is
WHITE.
Goodies for your tummy's delight.

? **What white veggie is shown to the right?**
ANSWER: Cauliflower

That veggie is good for Blake's _____ .
ANSWER: Stomach

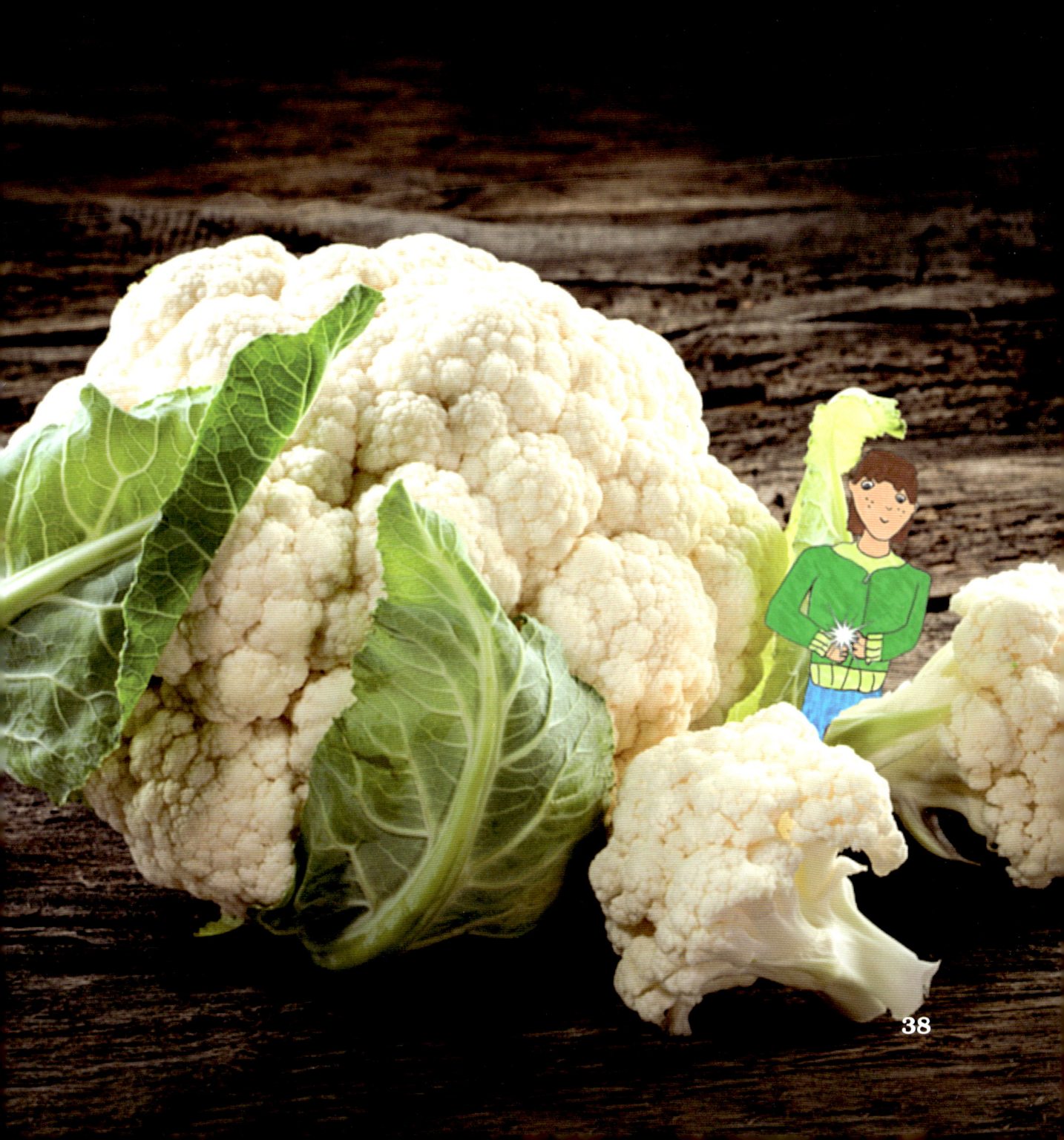

39

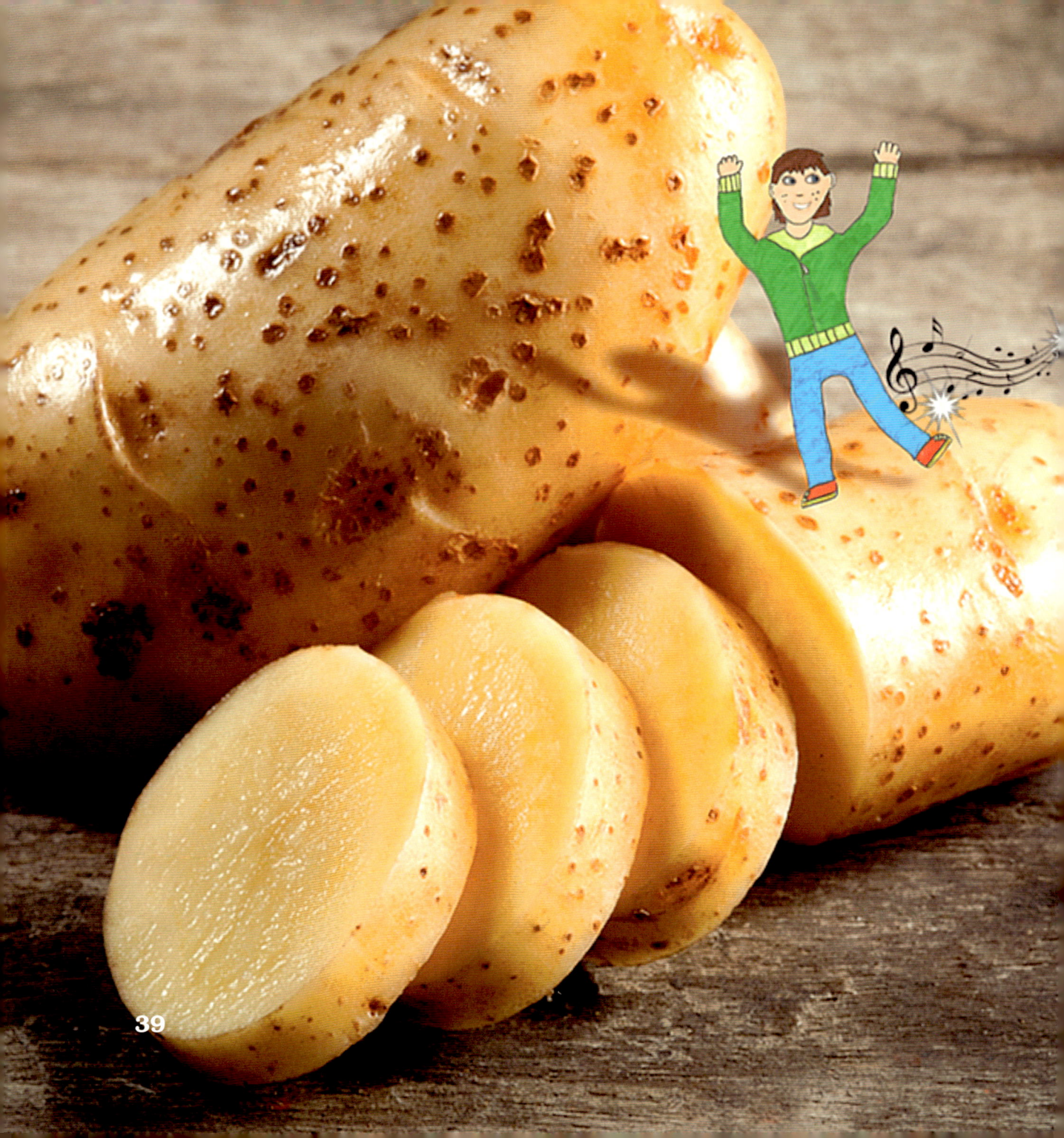

Eat **WHITE** foods when given the chance. They'll make you jump and sing and dance!

? **What white veggies are shown to the left?**
ANSWER: Potatoes

Do those veggies make Blake SLOW or GO?
ANSWER: GO!

[?] **What are some other WHITE fruits and veggies?**

ANSWER: Onions, turnips, mushrooms, jicama

[?] **Is Blake at the end of the path?**

ANSWER: Yes!

You helped Blake reach the pot of gold!

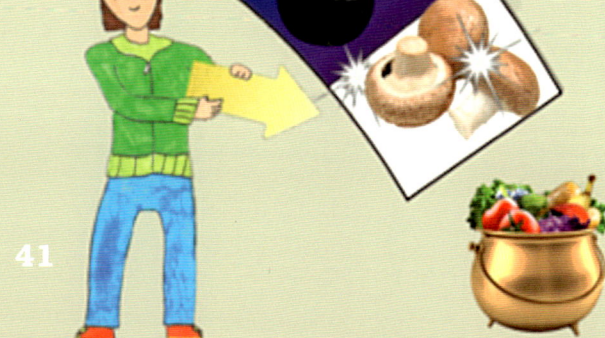

42

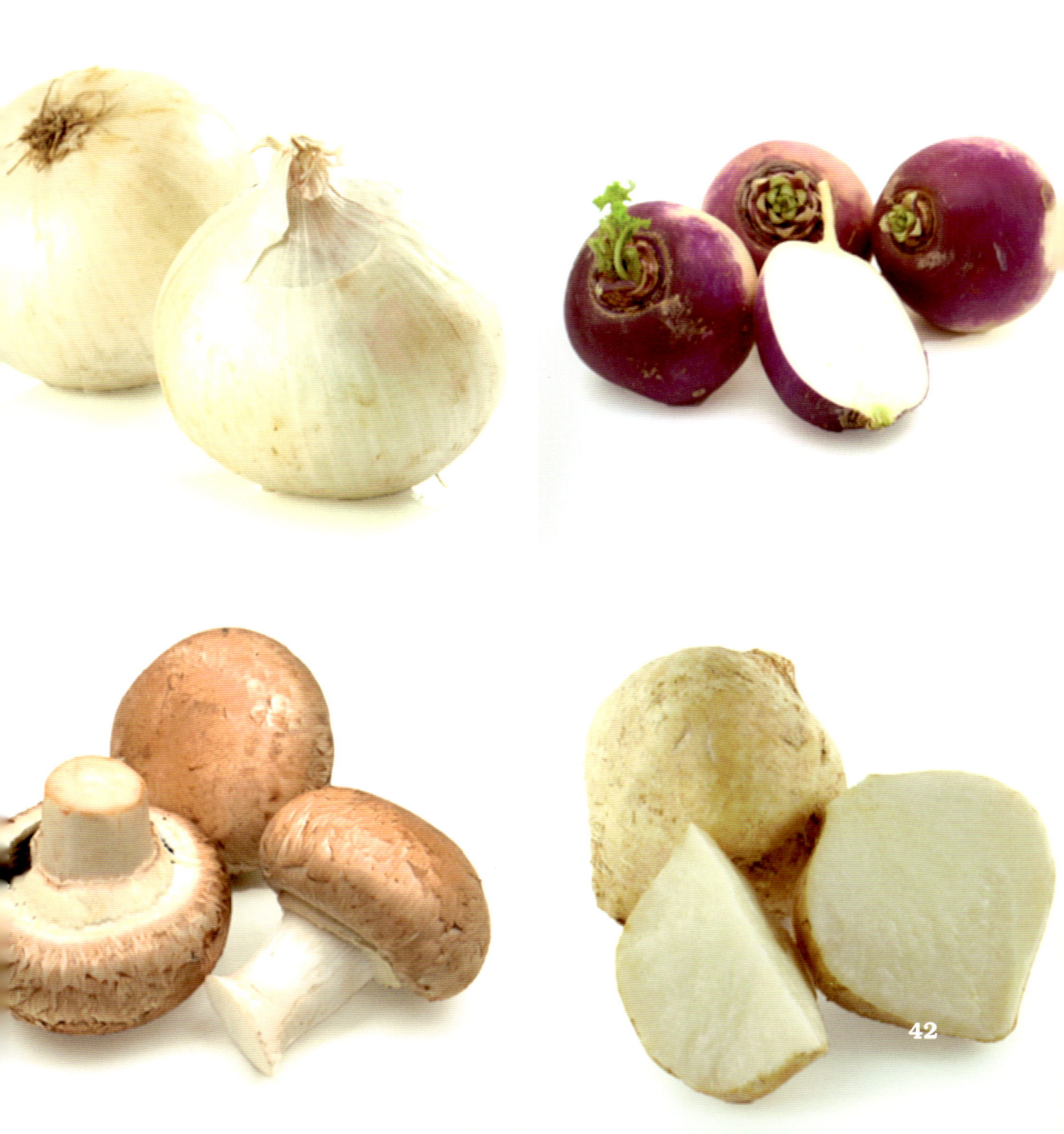

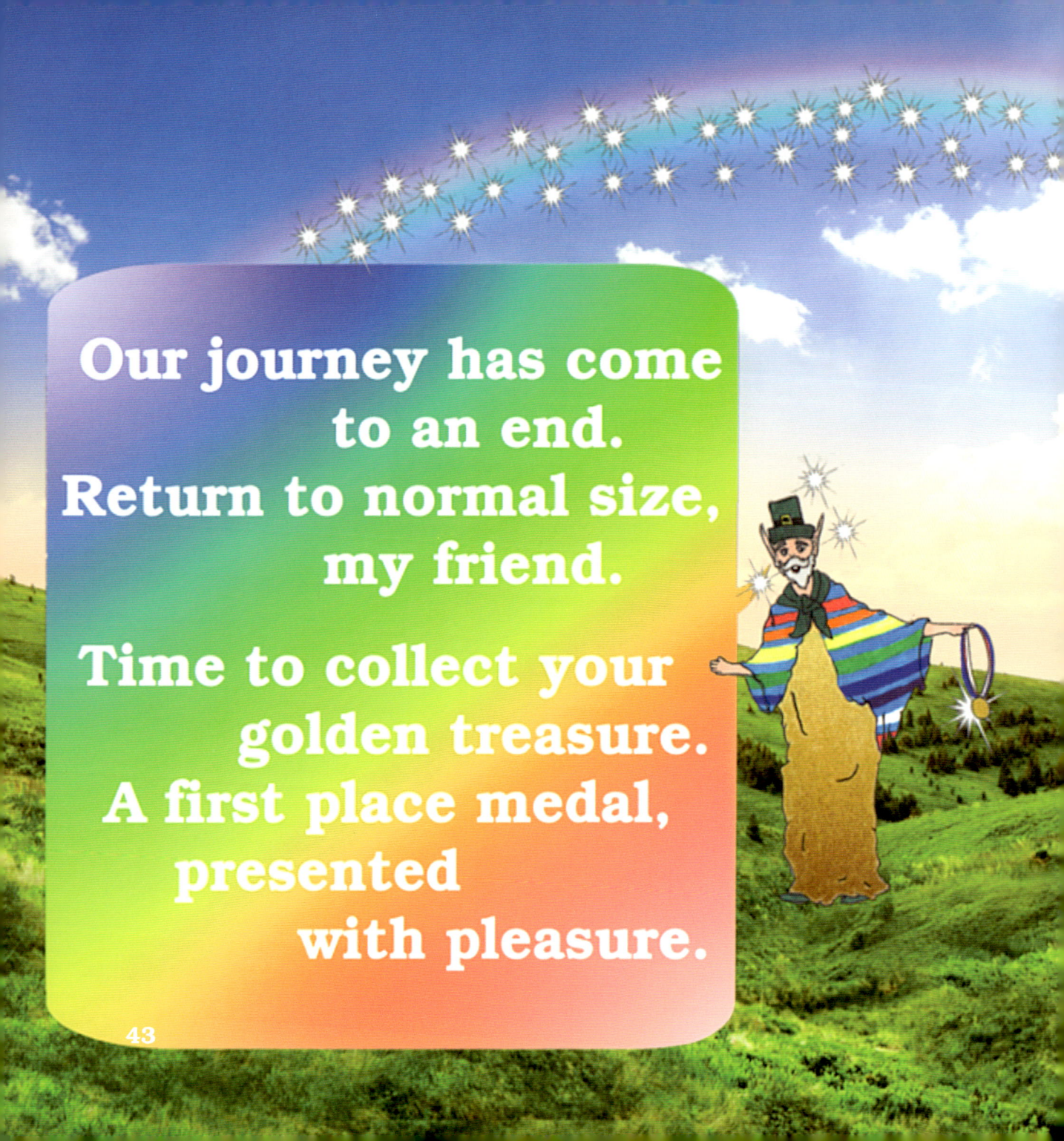

Our journey has come
to an end.
Return to normal size,
my friend.

Time to collect your
golden treasure.
A first place medal,
presented
with pleasure.

44

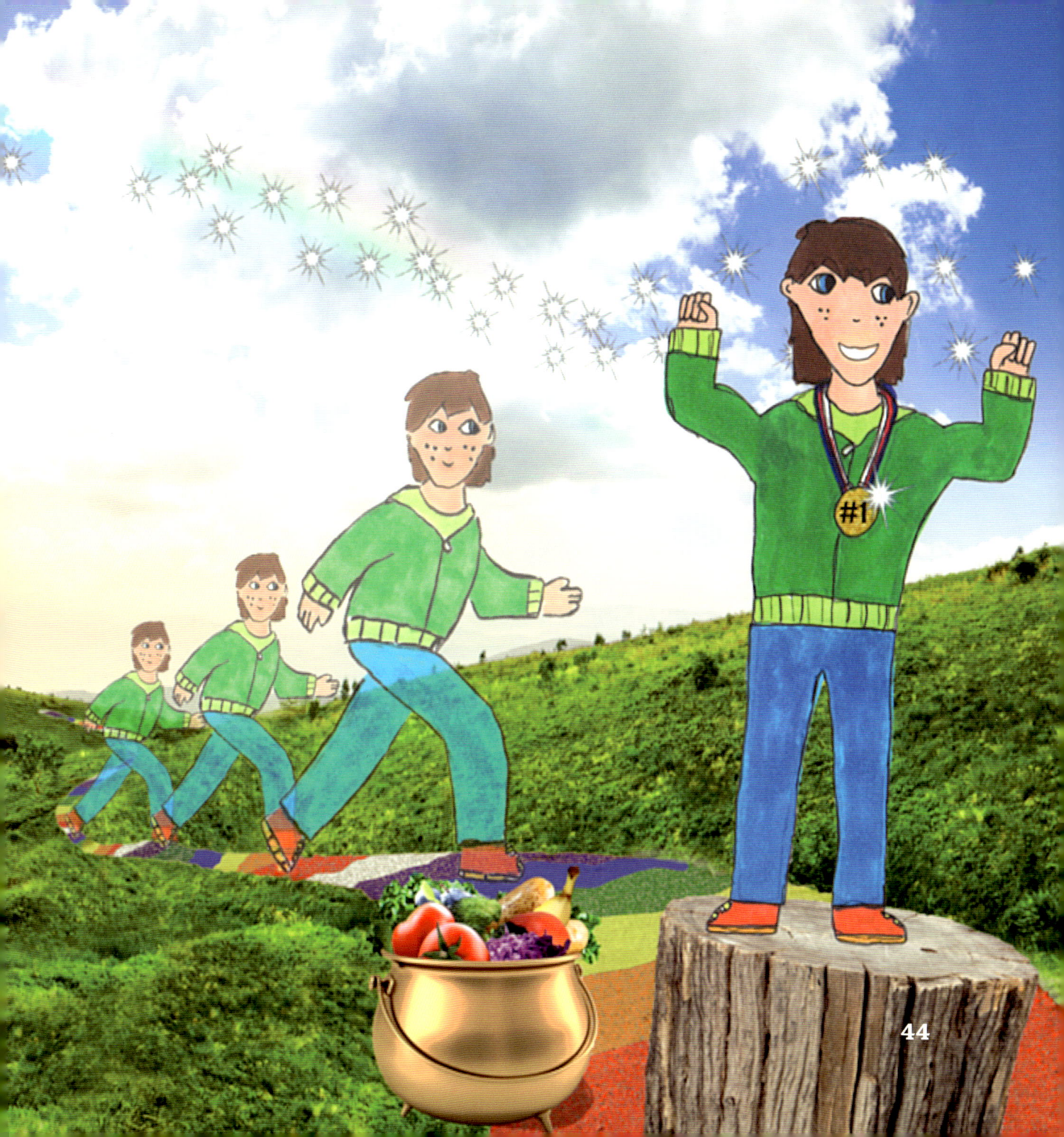

Inside YOU is all you seek.
A nourished body isn't tired and weak.

Eat fruits and veggies, then you play!
At least five servings every day.

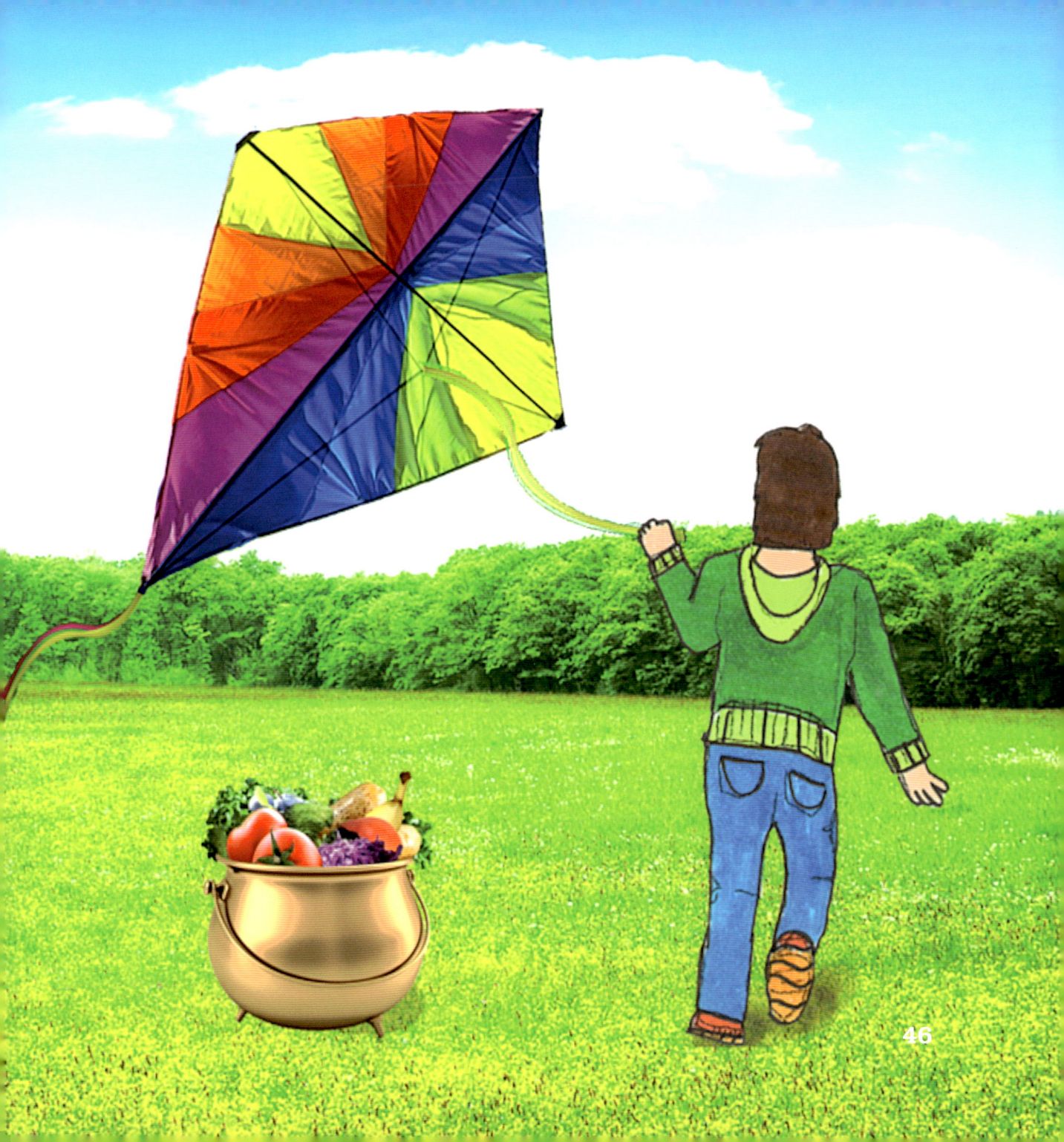

47

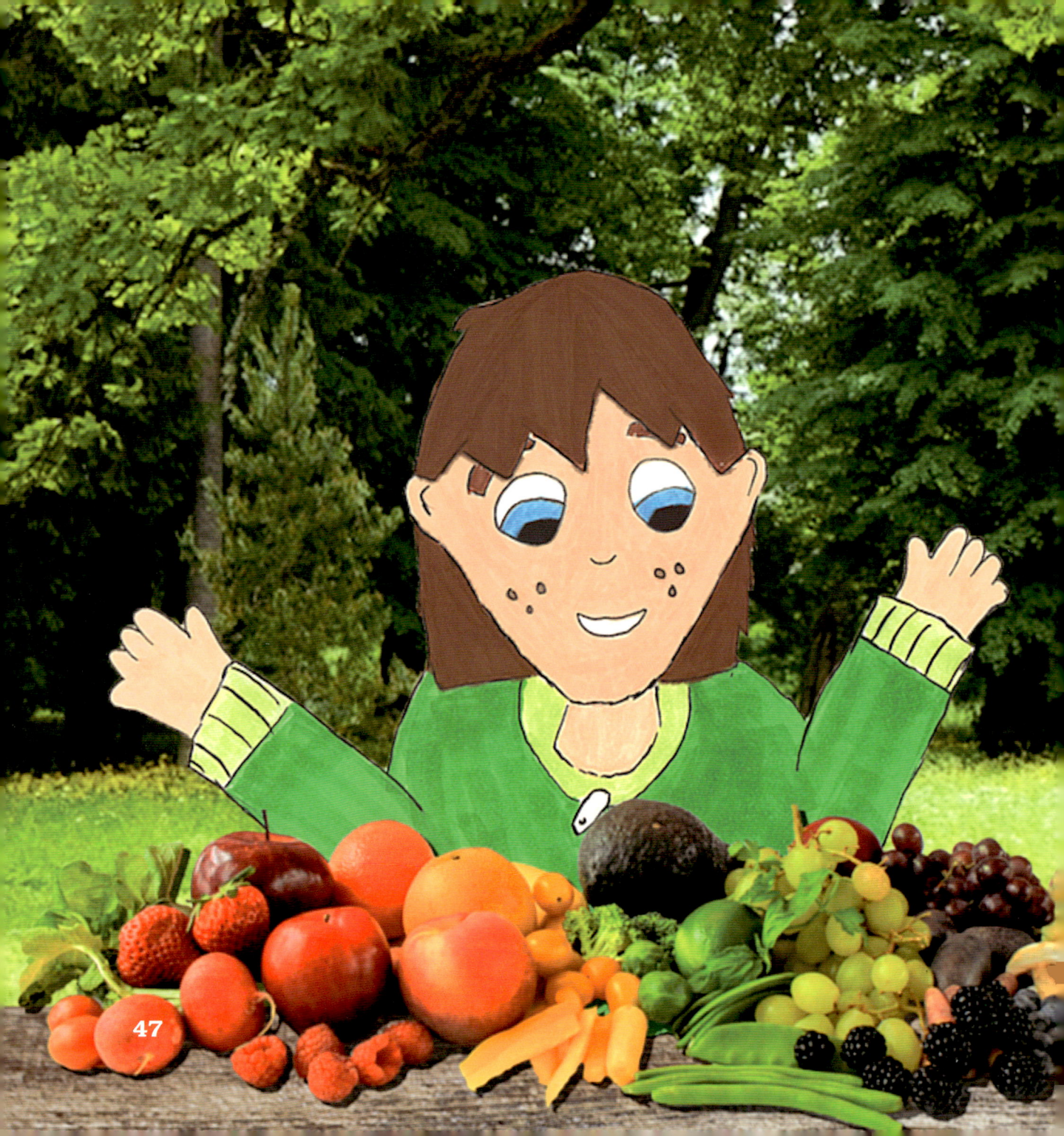

A pot of gold is in everyone.

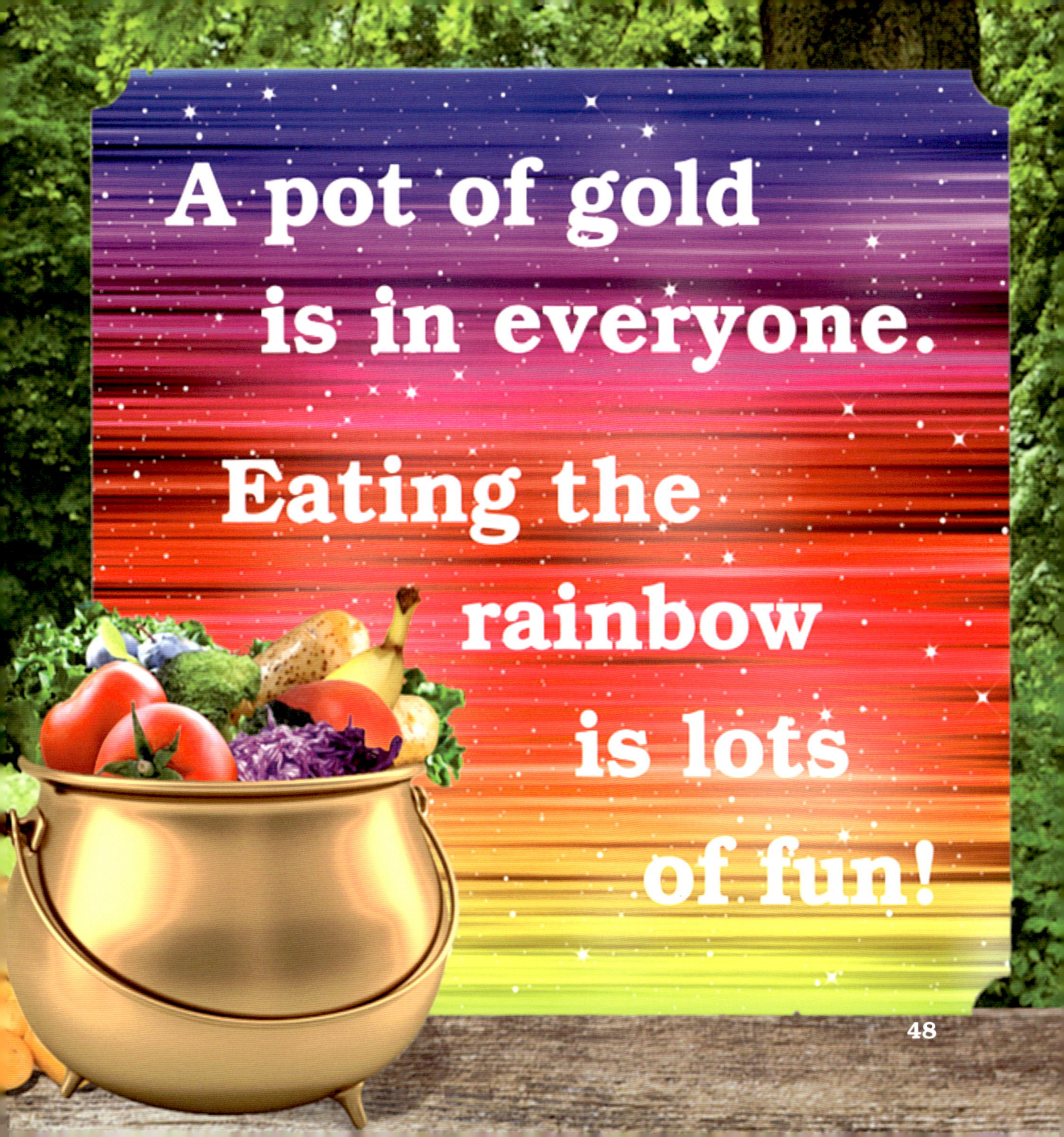

Eating the rainbow is lots of fun!

ABOUT THE AUTHOR

Kathryn Kemp Guylay is a certified nutritional counselor, speaker, writer, and coach with a master's degree in business. She is not afraid to dress up as a vegetable to visit schools and organizations on a national basis to get kids (and adults!) inspired to try new healthy foods. As the founder of the non-profit organization Nurture, Healthy Kids Ideas Exchange and Make Wellness Fun, Kathryn is on a mission to improve the health of our nation in a fun, action-oriented way.

Kathryn is the author of the award-winning and bestselling adult book on wellness, Mountain Mantras: Wellness and Life Lessons from the Slopes (September 2015).

Check the book out at the link:
www.mountainmantras.com

ABOUT THE ILLUSTRATOR

Illustrator **Alexander ("Alex") Guylay** attends middle school at Community School in Sun Valley, Idaho. Alex knows how to fuel his body for all of the activities he enjoys, including alpine skiing, Nordic skiing, playing hockey, mountain biking, and hiking. Alex has found inspiration for his illustrations from artists Jake Parker, Alan Blackwell, Matthew Armstrong, and -of course- Cara Frost.

ABOUT THE ARTISTIC TEAM

Art Director **Cara Frost** is a K-8 Art Educator at Community School in Sun Valley, Idaho, where she pursues her passion for education through art exploration, process, and instinct. She continues to develop her own style of art through ceramic sculpture, painting, stained glass, and the love of doodling.

Designer **Colleen Quindlen** has a diverse background in science, arts, health, and fitness. She is able to mix her technical mindset with creativity to help find solutions in a variety of projects. She currently lives in the beautiful mountains of Idaho and enjoys mountain biking, hiking, and playing in the snow with her boyfriend and their three dogs.

We've created a downloadable Blake (available at GiveItaGoEataRainbow.com) that you can color and cut out. Take a picture with Blake with your next healthy meal or snack and post it with #BlakeEatsaRainbow. Our "Flat Blake" is about building a broad community around eating healthy food and having fun!

Kids love a tangible treasure for their adventures. To allow all readers to celebrate their own journey when eating the colors, we've created a downloadable "first place medal" that you can also find at GiveItaGoEataRainbow.com.

We all agree that it takes a village to create an awesome book, and we are grateful to so many people who helped us on this project. Please see this link for our community of helpers.

www.healthysolutionsofsv.com/give-eat-rainbow-acknowledgements/

HEALTH BENEFITS OF FRUITS AND VEGGIES

RED fruits and veggies, such as tomatoes, peppers, and beets, contain lycopene. Lycopene has anti-inflammatory properties that are beneficial to the cardiovascular system.

ORANGE and YELLOW fruits and veggies, such as peppers, carrots, and sweet potatoes, are high in Vitamin A and Vitamin C. Vitamin A is especially important for eye development. Vitamin C is helpful in strengthening the immune system.

GREEN veggies, such as spinach, chard, and kale, contain calcium. Calcium is a mineral that is vital to the teeth and skeletal system (bones). Other GREEN fruits and veggies, such as broccoli, cucumbers, and lettuce, include B vitamins (including folate), critical micronutrients for optimal mental function.

BLUE and PURPLE fruits and veggies, such as blueberries, blackberries, and eggplant, are especially high in antioxidants. Antioxidants are powerful overall health boosters and are important for memory and healthy aging.

WHITE fruits and veggies, such as potatoes, mushrooms, and jicama, contain potassium and fiber. Fiber is extremely beneficial to the digestive system. Potassium is a mineral that, along with sodium and other minerals, allows the body to maintain electrolyte balance.